HAYFEVER

Dr Mark Payne is a General Practitioner working in Solihull who has been practising Environmental Medicine since 1979. He has a second career as a writer and a broadcaster making frequent radio and TV appearances and regularly producing articles for a wide variety of magazines and newspapers including a weekly column in the *Birmingham Post*.

HAYFEVER

HOW TO BEAT HAYFEVER
— PERMANENTLY

DR MARK PAYNE

Thorsons
An Imprint of HarperCollinsPublishers

Thorsons
An Imprint of HarperCollins*Publishers*
77–85 Fulham Palace Road,
Hammersmith, London W6 8JB

First published by Thorsons 1993 as
How to Beat Hayfever
This edition 1998

1 3 5 7 9 10 8 6 4 2

A catalogue record for this book
is available from the British Library

ISBN 0 7225 3630 5

Printed in Great Britain by
Caledonian International Book Manufacturing Ltd, Glasgow

TO LYNN

CONTENTS

ACKNOWLEDGEMENTS

Many people have at some time in their life nurtured a wish to write a book and see their name in print. However, despite the enormous advantages of word processors and electronic manipulation of text, relatively few books are completed. This is probably because of the colossal amount of time, energy and effort required to convert the initial thoughts into the finished product. You will get some idea of the volume of typing involved when I list those helping in the preparation of this manuscript, who include Jane Franklin, Nicki Lawrence, Liz Connor, Donna Jackson and Margaret Shepheard.

However, even more important than the physical help with manipulating the words is the encouragement, support and enthusiasm of my many good friends and family. They constantly supply me with new ideas and energy, and often step into the breach at short notice to help me out of a fix. My thanks go to Fabienne Alsing and Jeff Brinkley at the Alternative Medicine Centre, Milky John Currivan, Nellie, Vera, Audrey, Margot and Nora Gardner, Lola and Eddie Holland, Des and Sheila Martin, my Socratic teacher Rolph Norfolk, Eric and Margaret Payne, and my media advisors Roy and Virginia Ronnie. On a professional level I am indebted to Dr Norman Bertenshaw, Dr Jean Monro, and Professor Bill Rea.

Finally, none of this would have been worth doing without my family, who are Kelly, David and John, and my very special wife Lynn.

FOREWORD

This book has three objectives. The first is to explain how hayfever is caused. The second is to give you, the reader, simple practical measures which you can follow to get rid of the underlying causes. If you follow the recommendations of this book faithfully, then your hayfever could disappear completely, and it is very likely that your nose and eye symptoms will be reduced.

The third objective is to introduce you to the emerging science of Environmental Medicine which is able to offer most people:

- a feeling of positive well being
- an increase in energy level
- an improvement in concentration and memory
- a relatively easy way to get down to ideal weight
- a way to sleep well at night and wake up refreshed
- a way to control and sometimes cure common allergic illness like eczema, asthma, migraine and colitis.

It almost sounds too good to be true, but all Environmental Medicine does is give your body the best chance to put itself right in a world that is far from right.

The fundamental belief of Environmental Medicine is that the natural state of your body is health and if you're ill then it usually means that you're making a mistake with some part of your lifestyle: your diet, your job, your housing, your hobbies or your social situation. Environmental Medicine looks at all these areas in order to identify the factors that may be giving you the problem. When adverse factors are removed and adequate vitamins and mineral supplements given, the disease process can often be reversed with a return to positive health.

Environmental Medicine has five basic tenets. Although conventional medicine claims to follow some of these principles, in Environmental Medicine they are applied in a completely committed way.

THE HOLISTIC PRINCIPLE

In common with other forms of alternative medicine, Environmental Medicine comes to a diagnosis on the basis of the *total symptom picture* rather than looking merely at one organ. It then produces a treatment plan based on your lifestyle (diet, occupation, housing, hobbies and social situation). In contrast, conventional medicine has a much narrower approach and tends to home in on one symptom. Most of the effort is spent investigating a *single* organ to come to a diagnosis. Once a diagnosis has been made, the treatment is usually to take drugs for that single organ and there is little attention to the rest of the body and lifestyle.

THE PREVENTIVE PRINCIPLE

Environmental Medicine hopes to *prevent* illnesses from occurring or else treat them at a very early stage by removing the environmental causes of those illnesses. The majority of chronic diseases are at least partially **predictable**. They occur due to an error of lifestyle, e.g. a junk-food diet, exposure to chemicals at work, smoking, excess drinking, housing or hobbies filled with environmental hazards or a stressful home life. However, most disease processes are reversible if caught early. The body has an amazing ability to heal itself providing that the errors of lifestyle are removed. In order to get better, positive lifestyle change is essential.

THE PATIENT-POWER PRINCIPLE

Information is power, and the quality of your decisions is dependent on the quality of your information. A fundamental level of Environmental Medicine is to give you far more information, and therefore control, over your own health. Most of Environmental Medicine does not require the use of any drugs or medication; rather, the removal of all environmental factors causing illness. In many cases, a dramatic improvement in your health can be achieved by making these changes in your lifestyle. Environmental Medicine does, however, require **active** patient participation so that you take responsibility for your own health. This means altering your lifestyle to get rid of disease-promoting factors rather than just expecting to pop a pill.

THE RESOURCE MANAGEMENT PRINCIPLE

The basis of Environmental Medicine is the sensible management of the individual's limited resources to try to gain the best possible health. Environmental Medicine is seeking to reverse the alarming finding that people with fewer resources (time, money, education, family support), die younger and suffer from more illnesses. If the *existing* knowledge about disease-causing factors and their treatment is properly used, then better health and life expectancy is likely to follow.

THE SOCIAL CHANGES PRINCIPLE

Most health-related problems in the developed world are *political* rather than technological. The technologies to give the population clean food and water supply, sanitation, education, reasonable housing, transport and work conditions have been available since Roman times. It has taken 2,000 years for the political system to advance sufficiently to make these facilities commonly available in the western world. Radical improvements in health care will not occur until there are improvements in the political and social system.

HOW TO USE THIS BOOK

The way to gain maximum benefit from this book is to read it from cover to cover. This may sound like stating the obvious; however, this book is based on a holistic approach in which you need to understand the overall plan before you pay attention to the individual details. The fundamental principle of this book is the revolutionary new concept of 'The Total Load'. In summary, this concept states that the natural condition of the body is health and illness occurs when the 'Total Load' of pollutants or 'neotoxins' exceeds the body's capacity to detoxify them. A further vital part of this theory is that the cause of most illnesses is multifactorial. In other words, these illnesses do not arise from just a single factor but usually are caused by a combination of factors arising from diet, occupation, housing, hobbies and social situation. This book outlines the major sources of problems in hayfever. Each chapter then proposes practical solutions to overcome the problems. No one chapter has all the answers, but the best results are obtained when all the individual measures are put together.

Although every attempt has been made to make this guide accurate, comprehensive and easy to understand, no book is a substitute for the experience and overview of a competent practitioner. If you find that your symptoms persist or deteriorate when using this book then it is vital to see a qualified health practitioner without delay. The practitioner will then be able to exclude a wide variety of major and minor diseases which may mimic hayfever.

Finally, by reading this book you are at least half the way along the road to getting better. By taking the trouble to study hayfever, you have already realized that you have a health problem and provided that you are prepared to make the lifestyle changes necessary to reverse the course of your disease, then you are likely to get better. Good Luck!

INTRODUCTION

Hayfever is misery . . . But it doesn't have to be.

An astounding 1 in 5 people in Britain, the USA and Australia suffer from hayfever at some time in their life and yet relatively little has been done to help them beat their condition. Even more surprisingly, hayfever is becoming a lot more common, despite the fact that the amount of airborne pollen is dropping. This explosion in the incidence of hayfever is being caused by the widespread pollution of air, food and water which has become an integral part of the 20th-century mode of living.

The planet Earth is now starting to pay us back for 150 years of almost complete disregard for the long-term effects of industrial and domestic pollution on the environment and human health. Can the situation be remedied, or are we all condemned to increasing suffering from allergic conditions like hayfever, declining health and even extinction?

The good news is that hayfever can be beaten, or at least controlled, by following the practical measures described in this book.

Part One explains the processes that causes your hayfever. Part Two explains how you can treat your hayfever, firstly by reviewing your life in order to identify all the factors contributing to the problem. Secondly, you learn how to reduce them as much as possible, with the minimum disruption to your life.

A big bonus of this approach is that for most of the followers it usually produces a dramatic improvement in general health, energy level, memory and concentration.

IDENTIFYING YOUR TYPE OF HAYFEVER

1

What Happens in Hayfever

BACK TO THE DRAWING BOARD!

In medicine, sometimes you wonder if the so-called experts really know what they're talking about. For instance, take the term 'hayfever' which is almost completely wrong. The 'hayfever' is not caused by hay (which has no pollen); nor is there a fever, but the term is certainly understandable, considering the most obvious symptoms of running and itching eyes and nose. Hayfever is, in fact, an abnormal response or allergy (from the Greek *allos* meaning other, *ergon* meaning work or reaction) that some previously sensitized people show to pollen.

WHAT IS THE INCIDENCE OF HAYFEVER?

Hayfever is very common in the western world. During a typical hayfever season, it affects about 10 per cent of the population. That means that about 6 million people in Britain, and about 25 million people in the USA, are affected every year. To give you some idea of its importance, it is the only disease for which there are daily bulletins on the TV, radio and in the newspapers: these give a forecast of the pollen count, as a predictor of the likely severity of the disease. Hayfever usually starts between the age of 5 and 10 years and is rare in babies and old people. It reaches its peak incidence between 15 and 25 years. The symptoms are seasonal, occurring in June and July, especially at the end of June and the beginning of July, when the pollen count is at its highest.

Over the past few years, it has started to be realized that there is a very strong association between pollution and hayfever. Hayfever was first described in 1819, when the blue touch paper of the industrial revolution had just been lit. Although true hayfever cannot occur without pollen, we have, at present, the paradox of dropping pollen levels but increasing incidence of hayfever. This trend has become particularly obvious over the last 30 years. Table 1.1 shows the cumulative pollen level in June, which has been dropping over the past 30 years, compared with the incidence of hayfever, which has been increasing over the past 30 years.

Table 1.1: Hayfever prevalence compared with pollen count

Year	June total pollen count	Estimated prevalence of hayfever
1962	4,000	3%
1965	3,000	5%
1970	2,000	10%
1975	2,000	15%
1981	1,500	20%

The prevalence of hayfever is the *total* number of people suffering from the disease. This is not to be confused with the incidence, which is the number of *new* cases occurring in the year in question. The July total pollen count between 1962 and 1981 was fairly constant at 1,500. The severity of a hay fever season is assessed by the cumulative pollen count over June and July. If the total pollen count is over 5,000 then the season is said to be severe. If the total is 5,000 to 4,000 then the season is said to be moderate, and if the count is less than 4,000 than the season is said to be light.

The factors that have caused the pollen count to drop over the past 30 years are:

- an increased amount of grass that is turned into silage. (Silage is cut in May before pollen is released.)
- increased planting of timothy and rye grass, which release less pollen than the previous favourite, cocksfoot grass.

Symptoms of classical hayfever

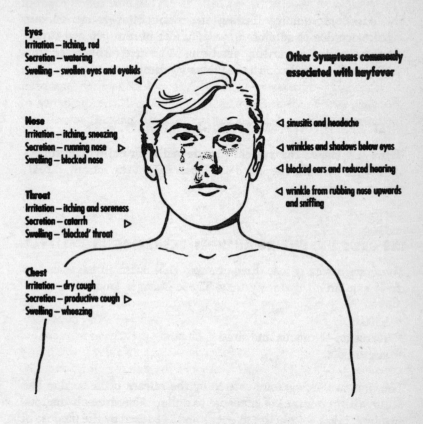

Eyes
Irritation – itching, red
Secretion – watering
Swelling – swollen eyes and eyelids

Other Symptoms commonly associated with hayfever

Nose
Irritation – itching, sneezing
Secretion – running nose
Swelling – blocked nose

◁ sinusitis and headache

◁ wrinkles and shadows below eyes

◁ blocked ears and reduced hearing

◁ wrinkle from rubbing nose upwards and sniffing

Throat
Irritation – itching and soreness
Secretion – catarrh
Swelling – 'blocked' throat

Chest
Irritation – dry cough
Secretion – productive cough
Swelling – wheezing

Figure 1.1: Symptoms of Hayfever

However, the single most important factor that has caused the incidence of hayfever to rise is:

- Reduced air quality. During the same 30 year period, air pollution due to sulphur dioxide, oxides of nitrogen and ozone has increased a startling six times. The main source of this increased air pollution is car exhaust fumes.

WHAT ARE THE TYPICAL SYMPTOMS OF HAYFEVER?

Figure 1.1 shows the typical picture of hayfever, which affects mainly the eyes and nose, and to a lesser extent the mouth, throat, ears and chest.

THE BASIC UNDERLYING CHANGES OCCURRING IN HAYFEVER

There are basically just three changes that occur in hayfever and these explain all the symptoms. These changes are:

- irritation
- secretion of mucus and fluid
- swelling.

The first two changes are caused by the release of histamine and occur within minutes of exposure to pollen. The third change, the swelling, takes 4-12 hours to occur and is caused by the process of inflammation which is set off by the release of many complex chemicals called mediators. Table 1.2 shows how the three changes are able to cause all the symptoms of hayfever.

Table 1.2: Changes in hayfever

CHANGE	EYES	NOSE	CHEST
Irritation	Itching Red	Itching Sneezing	Dry cough
Secretion	Watering Clear fluid	Runny nose; clear discharge	Productive rattling cough + wheezing
Swelling	Swelling eye lining	Blocked nose	Wheezing increases

WHY DOES HAYFEVER OCCUR?

Hayfever is an example of the commonest type of allergic reaction that takes place in the body. It occurs because the body's defence mechanism against infections, the immune system, becomes confused and reacts inappropriately to plant pollens (from trees, grasses or weeds), which are mistaken for dangerous invaders. The allergic reaction occurring in the body can be summarized in figure 1.2. Once you understand this fairly straightforward process, then it will also become clear how hayfever can be prevented or its symptoms, at least, reduced by blocking the process at one or more points.

The situation in real life is that the grass pollen becomes airborne and lands on the mucous membrane of the eyes, nose, throat or lungs. These mucous membranes are moist and contain enzymes, which strip off the outer protective coat of the pollen. Consequently the water-soluble proteins in the pollen dissolve and interact with the immune system of the body.

In people with a normal immune system there is no reaction and that is the end of the story. But in those with a malfunctioning immune system, the protein in the pollen sets off an allergic response that causes the symptoms of hayfever. The sequence of

Figure 1.2: Reactions Occurring in Classical Hayfever

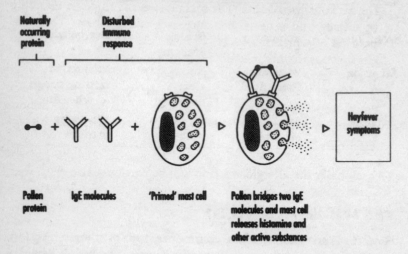

events after the pollen lands on the mucous membranes of a
hayfever sufferer is as follows:

- the pollen is 'recognized' by the branched end of two identical
  pollen-specific antibody molecules (called IgE). This causes an
  effect called 'bridging'.
- the other end of the IgE molecule has already attached itself
  to a receptor site on the surface of a special cell in the blood
  called a mast cell. This is the final part of an effect called
  'priming'.
- The 'bridging' between two IgE molecules causes the mast cell
  to release a substance called histamine, which causes the
  'immediate reaction' and after a few hours other substances are
  synthesized that cause the 'delayed reaction'.
- The histamine has two effects, both of which commence within
  minutes of pollen exposure; provided that there is no further
  exposure, they wear off in about three hours. The first effect is

irritation caused by a local action of histamine on the cells of the mucous membrane. The second effect is that the secretion of mucus and other fluids increases many times. This outpouring of secretions occurs because the tiny blood vessels in the mucous membranes suddenly become much more leaky and let out lots of serum from the blood.

- The other substances which cause the 'delayed reaction' act much more slowly and cause all the usual signs of inflammation, which are redness swelling, heat, pain and loss of function.

Occasionally the allergic reaction will be particularly severe, then it may give rise to a life-threatening condition known as 'anaphylaxis' or 'anaphylactic shock'. This severe type of reaction can occur when a protein like pollen or fish is injected into or eaten by a highly allergic individual.

In anaphylaxis, large amounts of histamine are suddenly released from the mast cells. In seconds very obvious symptoms affecting all the major systems occur, including

- Heart and blood vessels: severe drop in blood pressure and very fast, faint pulse.
- Lungs: wheezing, shortness of breath, asthma, patient may go blue, due to lack of oxygen reaching lungs and blood.
- Brain: unconsciousness, due to low blood pressure and reduced circulating oxygen.

NB: If you suspect a severe allergic reaction you must get medical help *immediately*.

WHICH PLANT POLLENS ARE MOST LIKELY TO CAUSE HAYFEVER?

Hayfever can be caused by tree, grass or weed pollens. Table 1.3 lists the majority of plants that may cause hayfever in Britain.

Table 1.3: Plants that may cause hayfever

SPRING

TREES	TREES (cont.)	GRASSES	WEEDS
Alder	Pine	Annual	Capeweed
Ash	Plane	meadow	Clover
Beech	Poplar	grass	Dandelion
Birch	Privet	Barley grass	Paterson's
Elder	Sycamore	Prairie grass	curse
Elm	Willow	Rye grass	Plantain
Hawthorn	Yew	Sweet vernal	Wattle
Hazel		Wheat	Wheat
Horse		Wild oats	Wild
chestnut		Yorkshire fog	mustard
Maple			
Oak			

SUMMER

TREES	GRASSES	GRASSES (cont.)	WEEDS
Maple	Annual	False oat	Clover
Olive	meadow	Fescue	Dandelion
Pine	grass	Foxtail	Dock
Privet	Bent	Maize	Mulberry
	Broom	Rhodes	Nettles
	Canary grass	Rye grass	Plantain
	Cocksfoot	Sweet vernal	Sorrel
	Couch grass	Timothy	Wild
	Dogstail	Veldt	mustard
		Yorkshire fog	

LATE SUMMER

GRASSES	GRASSES (cont.)	WEEDS	FLOWERS
Annual meadow grass	Canary grass	Dandelion	Pellitory
Bent	Cocksfoot	Fat hen	Golden rod
Bermuda grass	Couch grass	Heather (wild)	Lupin
	False oat	Mugwort	
	Maize	Nettles	
	Rye grass	Plantain	

AUTUMN AND WINTER

TREES	GRASSES
Cedar	Annual meadow grass
Hazel	
Yew	Wild oats

Although there are some exceptions to the rule, in general the flowering seasons of different types of plants in Britain are as follows:

- tree pollen - February to May
- grass pollen - May to July
- weed pollen - July to October
- cereals - July and August

More specific information about the times of flowering are given in the following chapters.

In Britain by far the biggest problem is caused by grass pollen. However, the major culprit causing hayfever varies quite a bit from country to country. Tree pollens tend to be more of a problem in countries with limited rainfall.

Important Causes of Hayfever by Country

COUNTRY	POLLEN FROM	HAYFEVER MONTH
North America	Ragweed	Aug/Sept
Scandinavia	Birch tree	May/June
UK	Grasses	June/July
Alps	Birch	March/April
Mediterranean	Mulberry pollen & olive tree	April/May
Japan	Cedar tree	March/April
Australia	Wattle	September

WHAT FACTORS DECIDE WHETHER A PLANT POLLEN IS LIKELY TO CAUSE HAYFEVER?

Theoretically, any pollen could be the cause of hayfever. However, for a plant to be a culprit that commonly causes hayfever there are three main requirements.

High Air Pollen Concentration

Pollen needs to be released in large amounts from each plant, and that plant needs to be common in that area. The ragweed fulfils these two requirements. In the season each plant may release up to one million pollen grains daily. It has been estimated that a square mile of this plant would release sixteen tons of pollen in a season. The ragweed has a very wide distribution in America, especially on the west coast where it grows both on cultivated land and on wasteland. A hayfever sufferer will react to a concentration of 50 pollen grains per cubic metre. During an average summer day, there may be as many as 200 pollen grains per cubic metre.

Easily Transported by the Wind

The pollen grains should be small and non-sticky, so that they can travel a considerable distance on the wind. Pollen varies in size from 20–200 microns (1 micron = 1/1000 of a millimetre), but most pollens causing hayfever are at the smaller end, between 20 and 40 microns in diameter. Ragweed pollen is easily windborne and has been found four hundred miles out to sea.

Able to Cause Allergy

The pollen must contain enough of the right sort of protein, which is able to set off an allergic reaction in a suitable individual. Pine trees are a good example of a low allergy pollen that does not cause hayfever, despite being present in very large amounts near pine forests and being able to travel considerable distances on the wind.

WHAT FACTORS AFFECT AIR POLLEN CONCENTRATION?

The biggest single factor affecting the pollen concentration is the weather. Although at any given location, pollen is released very reliably during the same week each year, there may be immense year to year variations. Grass pollen levels may vary by a factor of 2 to 3 from year to year, whereas tree pollen, especially that of birch, may vary by a factor of 15 from year to year. This is one explanation for the variation in severity of symptoms from year to year. As a general rule, the further away that you move from the equator, the later in the year that plants flower and pollinate. This northwards delay is noticeable even in Britain where plants on the south coast flower about a month before those in Scotland.

WHAT FACTORS MAKE HAYFEVER BETTER OR WORSE?

The two most important factors that affect the likelihood of hayfever are the weather (which governs pollen level) and air pollution.

Factors That Make Hayfever Worse

- Increased pollen count caused by:
    rain before season
    warm temperature
    sunshine
    slight to moderate wind
- Increased air pollution caused by:
    living in a city or near road/factory
    still air conditions
    fog/smog

Factors That Make Hayfever Better

- being indoors
- air conditioning and air filtration
- being in mountainous and seaside areas
- rain, especially fine rain
- low air pollution

THE IgE ANTIBODY

The IgE antibody is an essential component in the hayfever process. Its structure is shown in figure 1.3.

The IgE molecule is made of two pairs of identical paired chains. There are the light chains (shaded), which are attached by sulphur bonds to the heavy chains.

Although the IgE molecule is much too small to be seen by the eye or light microscope, it is known to be Y-shaped and the Fab end is highly selective and will react only with one pollen. It is this that makes the IgE molecule able to recognize only one specific protein and ignore all the rest. The recognition occurs after the white cells of the body have been exposed to that particular pollen, which is a very important process called 'priming'. If priming has not previously occurred then no hayfever reaction takes place.

Figure 1.3: The IgE molecule

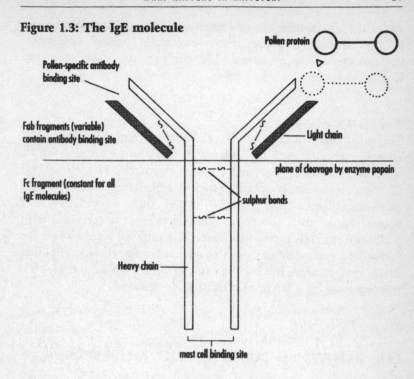

The Fc end of the molecule binds to the surface of the mast cell, each of which has approximately 300,000 receptor sites. The protein of the pollen reacts with the receptors on the Fab end of several IgE molecules causing 'bridging'. This bridging triggers an immediate release of histamine from granules in the mast cell followed later by other substances which cause the 'delayed response'.

Why IgE is Produced

The IgE antibody, together with a white cell called an *eosinophil*, have been developed by the body to combat invasion by intestinal parasites and worms. These parasites are much too large to be swallowed up by an individual white cell in the usual way that bacteria are killed. Instead, the parasite is recognized by the IgE molecule which then attracts the eosinophils. When stimulated by the allergic responses the eosinophils release poisonous substances, which are able to kill the parasite or at least stop further invasion.

The Mast Cell

The mast cell is a large white cell which is fundamental to the allergic response seen in hayfever. It has many granules which contain histamine. The name comes from the fact that their German discoverer thought that they were well-nourished cells and called them *mast zelle* (*mast* = food + *zelle* = cell). Hayfever cannot occur until the mast cells have become 'primed' with pollen-specific IgE antibodies which slot into the receptors on the membrane surface. Mast cells also respond to the amount of pollen in the environment. In a hayfever sufferer, the number of mast cells may increase by a factor of 8 during the season.

CAN 'HAYFEVER' BE CAUSED BY OTHER FACTORS?

Classical hayfever occurs only when the pollen to which the sufferer is sensitive is in the air. There are, however, several other types of biological material that can cause hayfever-like symptoms. These include:

- fungal spores (dealt with in more detail in chapter 5)
- house dust mite (dealt with in more detail in chapter 6)
- animal hairs (dealt with in more detail in chapter 6).

In order to decide which factor is most likely to be causing your hayfever-like symptoms, you should consult table 1.4. Don't forget to arm yourself first with details of times and places where the symptoms are best or worst.

Table 1.4: Time/Place Where Allergy is Worse and Likely Cause of 'Hayfever'

TIME OF YEAR/DAY WHEN ALLERGY IS WORSE	PLACE WHERE ALLERGY IS WORSE	CAUSE OF ALLERGY
February to May		Tree pollen
May to July	Outside, especially near fields & woods	Grass pollen
July to October		Weed pollen
July and August		Cereals
All year round with peak August to October	Outdoors in *damp* places & near water	Fungal spores
All year round with peak August to October	Indoors in *damp* places, e.g. bathrooms & basements and near water	Fungal spores
All year round with peak in winter	Indoors especially in old damp houses, near open water & underground streams	House dust mites
All year round with seasonal peak moulting season	Indoors especially near animal's sleeping place	Pet furs and feathers
In winter	Indoors	Any form of indoor pollution

IS IT HAYFEVER OR JUST A COLD?

There are major differences between hayfever or other form of allergic rhinitis and cold symptoms which are summarized in the following table. As a general rule, hayfever comes on much more suddenly, sneezing is common, and the discharge is watery and clear rather than yellow.

SYMPTOMS OF ALLERGIC RHINITIS	SYMPTOMS OF A 'COLD'
Sudden onset	More gradual onset
Frequent sneezing (often within seconds)	Sneezing rare
Clear watery discharge	Yellow discharge
Eyes also affected	Eyes usually spared

IS HAYFEVER INHERITED?

Hayfever, together with asthma and eczema, falls into a special category of allergy called atopy (Greek: literally out of place). If one of your parents suffers from atopic symptoms, then your likelihood of allergy is increased. If both parents suffer, then you have a much greater likelihood of suffering from allergy.

The factor causing the allergy to be inherited is probably a partial or complete enzyme deficiency giving rise to the allergic symptoms.

HEREDITY	ALLERGIC RISK
If neither parent is allergic	10-20 per cent
If either parent is allergic	30-50 per cent
If both parents are allergic	40-75 per cent

HOW CAN I TELL WHICH PARTICULAR POLLEN IS CAUSING MY HAYFEVER?

There are two commonly used ways to tell which pollen is causing your hayfever. They both depend on there being an increased level of specific IgE antibody in the blood.

The first is called the **prick test**. It is carried out by putting one drop of a pollen solution on the skin of the forearm. The skin is then carefully pricked, allowing a tiny amount of the pollen protein to penetrate the outermost layers of the skin. If there is an increased level of IgE to that particular pollen solution, then a small raised weal (which looks like a nettle sting) surrounded by a red flare will be produced.

This weal takes about five to ten minutes to form and the greater the reaction, the larger the weal and surrounding red flare. The weal is either scored on a scale from + to + + + + or else a ball point pen is used to trace accurately around the weal. Then the ink is lifted off using a piece of transparent sticky tape which can be stuck on the patient's notes as a permanent record. The prick test does not work properly if the patient has taken an antihistamine preparation in the 24 hours prior to the test.

The common battery of skin prick tests carried out include:

pollens
    early season flowering trees   grasses
    mid-season flowering trees   weeds
fungal mix(es)
animals
    cat   feather   horse
    dog   hamster   rabbit
house dust mite
positive control - containing histamine which produces standardized size weal for that individual
negative control - should produce no weal to ensure that patient does not react to glycerol base of test preparations

The second method to determine which pollen a patient is allergic to is a laboratory investigation called a **RAST test** (radio allergosorbent test). This test is very sensitive and is able to give a quantitative measure of the level of allergy to a specific pollen. It is, however, rather expensive and requires to be carried out in a laboratory specifically geared for the investigation.

The reason that the RAST test is so useful is that instead of just measuring the total IgE level, it is able to identify IgE for specific pollens like birch tree, cocksfoot grass, or ragweed. This gives a strong indication of the precise substances that the tested person is allergic to.

The RAST test is carried out in two stages. In the first stage the patient's blood is incubated with a panel of paper discs, each coated with a different pollen extract. If IgE specific to the pollen on the disc is present in the blood tested then the Fab end of the IgE antibody binds firmly to the disc. The disc is then washed to remove the non-bound IgE. The disc is then incubated with a non-specific anti-IgE antibody. This non-specific anti-IgE antibody reacts with the Fc end of any IgE molecule that has already bound to the pollen on the disc. The disc is once again washed to remove all non-bound antibodies. The amount of non-specific anti-IgE antibody can then be measured very accurately because it has previously been radioactively labelled. Consequently, the amount of pollen-specific IgE in the blood sample can be deduced very accurately.

HOW CAN HAYFEVER BE PREVENTED OR AT LEAST CONTROLLED?

The information which will help you to do this is contained in the following chapters but, since it is very helpful to have an overview of the complete picture, a summary of how to beat hayfever follows.

1 analyse your own hayfever problem
2 work out your own customized hayfever plan to:
   reduce your pollen exposure
   repair your immune system
   reduce your total load of pollutants
   take vitamin and mineral supplements
   use symptomatic treatment for any remaining problems

Figure 1.4: RAST test

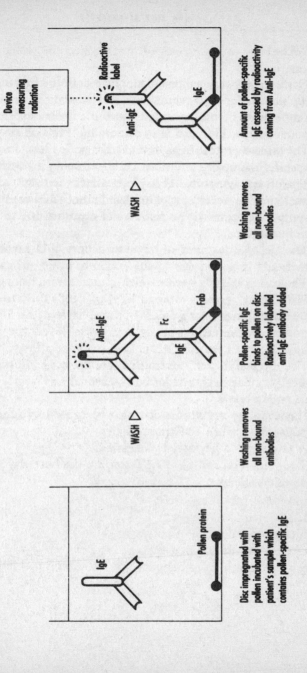

Disc impregnated with pollen incubated with patient's sample which contains pollen-specific IgE

WASH △

Washing removes all non-bound antibodies

Pollen-specific IgE binds to pollen on disc. Radioactively labelled anti-IgE antibody added

WASH △

Washing removes all non-bound antibodies

Amount of pollen-specific IgE assessed by radioactivity coming from Anti-IgE

IgE

Pollen protein

Anti-IgE

Fc

Fab

IgE

Device measuring radiation

Radioactive label

Anti-IgE

IgE

SUMMARY

- Hayfever is a very common allergic reaction, affecting 1 in 5 of the population in a typical hayfever season.
- Hayfever is becoming much more common despite dropping pollen levels. This is due to increasing levels of air pollution.
- The disease process in hayfever is that pollen reacts with pollen-specific antibodies and mast cells, releasing histamine.
- The classic symptoms of hayfever affect the eyes and nose and are irritation, secretions of fluid and mucus and swelling. These symptoms occur within minutes of exposure due to the action of histamine.
- The 'delayed reaction' of hayfever occurs 4–12 hours after the exposure to pollen due to the action of other substances.
- The pollen causing hayfever either comes from trees (in the UK, Feb to May), grasses (May to July) or weeds (July to Oct).
- the requirements for a pollen to cause hayfever are for a high air pollen concentration, easily transportable on the wind, and having pollen protein that is able to cause allergy.
- The biggest factor controlling pollen concentration is the weather. This accounts for both seasonal and hourly variations in pollen levels.
- Hayfever-like symptoms can also be caused by fungal spores, house dust mites and animal hairs.
- A tendency to hayfever is inherited.
- The prick test and the RAST test are the best way to confirm a pollen allergy.

2

Early Season Hayfever and Tree Pollens

It's very fortunate that most coniferous trees don't cause hayfever, or else the inhabitants of Scandinavia, for example, might find life very difficult. In fact, a relatively small proportion of British hayfever sufferers are susceptible to tree pollen; the tree pollen season is also shorter than that of grasses and weeds.

Tree pollen tends to cause problems in dry regions where rainfall is low and grass doesn't manage to grow very well. Some well-known tree pollen allergies include the silver birch in Scandinavia, olive trees around the Mediterranean, the prosoba tree in the Middle East, and the cedar tree in Japan.

The trees which are known to give hayfever problems in Britain are listed in table 2.1, but the main culprits include Alder, Beech, Birch, Elm, False Acacia, Hawthorn, Horse Chestnut, Hazel, Oak, Poplar, Plane and Willow.

The flowering (pollination) season of trees commonly causing hayfever is also shown in table 2.1.

For diagnosis of tree hayfever, it is helpful to divide trees into two groups: the early season pollinators (Jan to April) and the mid-season pollinators (May to June).

EARLY SEASON POLLINATORS

- Alder - pollinates February to March. Alder is common throughout Britain, growing in woods by lakes and streams and on waste ground.

Table 2.1: Tree Pollen Chart

Tree	Jan	Feb	Mar	Apr	May	Jun	Jul	Aug	Sep	Oct	Nov	Dec	Comments
Hazel	███	███	███	██									
Alder		███	███										
Elm		███	███										
Poplar		█	███	█									
Ash				███	███								
Willow				███	██								
Beech				███	██								
Birch				███	███								
Plane				███	██								
Oak				███	██								
Sycamore				███	███	██							
Hawthorne				█	███	█							
Horse Chestnut				█	███	█							
False Acacia					██								
Elder					███	██							

- Elm - pollinates February to March. Elm likes to grow in hedges and by roads although its numbers have been greatly reduced by the plague of Dutch Elm Disease. It is more common in the south of Britain.
- Hazel - pollinates January to April. Hazel likes to grow in woods and hedges.
- Poplar - pollinates late February to early April. Poplar likes to grow in wet areas. It is distributed throughout Britain.
- Willow - pollinates April to May. Willow likes to grow in wet areas, especially near streams, rivers and marshes.

MID-SEASON POLLINATORS

- Ash - pollinates April to May. Ash like to grow on chalky soils in the wetter parts of Britain.

- Beech – pollinates April to May. Beech grows mostly in southeast England and prefers chalky and limestone soils.
- Birch – pollinates April to May. Birch likes to grow in woods and heathland all over Britain. The Silver Birch is more common in southern England. In Scandinavia, birch pollen is one of the most common causes of hayfever.
- Elder – pollinates June to July, and likes to grow in woods and waste ground and along roadsides. It occurs throughout Britain and pollinates later than other trees.
- False Acacia – pollinates in June. False Acacia is not a natural inhabitant of Britain but is usually cultivated and may be planted in thickets.
- Hawthorn – pollinates May to June. Hawthorn likes to grow on acid and peaty soils and is planted extensively in hedgerows. It is common throughout England.
- Horse Chestnut – pollinates May and June. Horse chestnut likes to grow in woods with other hardwood trees. It occurs all over Britain.
- Oak – pollinates April and May. Oak likes to grow in woods and hedgerows, particularly in loam and clay soils. It grows throughout Britain.
- Plane/London Plane – pollinates April and May. Plane is not a native of Britain but has been extensively planted in cities, probably because it is resistant to pollution.
- Sycamore – pollinates April to June. Sycamore likes to grow in woods and hedges. It is distributed throughout Britain.

TESTS FOR TREE POLLENS

You may well be able to determine which trees are causing your problems by observation. If you're not very good at identifying trees, then find a book or a botanist friend and make a note of the trees growing in your garden. Don't forget to look over the fence and see which trees your neighbours have growing, since pollens are no respecters of boundaries. Note the prevailing wind direction, since you will receive proportionally more pollen from trees that are upwind and less from ones that are downwind. You can find out which way the wind is blowing by licking your index finger and holding it up in the air. The side that feels cold indicates the direction the wind is blowing from.

Skin prick testing and RAST testing (see page 33) are very useful to establish exactly which tree you react to. It's important that you haven't taken an antihistamine preparation in the 24 hours before a prick test, since this may reduce your reaction and the accuracy of the test. RAST testing is carried out on a sample of your blood and is unaffected by antihistamine medication.

HOW CAN I CURE MY TREE POLLEN ALLERGY?

You will need to read the rest of this book, particularly Part Two. As a general rule a broad approach, in which you try to reduce all the factors contributing to the hayfever, is usually the most successful. In the worst cases of tree hayfever, this could mean cutting down one or more trees that affect you, especially if they are close to your home. In Britain you may need planning permission if the tree is large and, if the problem is severe, you may even consider moving house.

3

Main Season Hayfever and Grass Pollen

Grasses are the success story of the plant world. There are over 10,000 species that grow widely on all continents. It is estimated that grasses cover a staggering 20 per cent of the total land surface of the world. When most people talk of hayfever, they usually mean the condition caused by grass pollen.

In temperate zones in the northern hemisphere, the grass hayfever season starts in May and runs to the end of July. In the UK it is at its peak, causing the maximum disruption, during the period when schools and colleges have their exams.

The major culprits causing grass hayfever are Bent, Broom, Cocksfoot and Dogstail, Fescue, Foxtail, Meadowgrass, Ryegrass, Timothy, Vernal and Yorkshire Fog. The pollination periods are shown in table 3.1.

- Bent - pollinates June to August. Bent likes to grow in acid soils such as heaths, moorlands. It is widely distributed throughout Britain.
- Broom - pollinates June and July. Broom likes to grow in woods and shady places. It grows throughout Britain except in the north of Scotland.
- Cocksfoot and Dogstail - these grasses pollinate twice. They have a major yield in May and June with a lesser yield in June and July. Overall, these are very heavy pollinators and consequently a major cause of hayfever. These grasses like to grow in fields, woods and on waste ground.
- Fescue - pollinates in June. Fescue likes to grow in meadows. It has a wide distribution throughout Britain, though not in the north of Scotland.

Table 3.1: Grass Pollen Chart

Tree	Jan	Feb	Mar	Apr	May	Jun	Jul	Aug	Sep	Oct	Nov	Dec	Comments
Vernal				▬	▬	▬							
Foxtail				▬	▬	▬							
Meadowgrass					▬	▬	▬						
Cocksfoot					▬	▬	▬	▬					
Dogtail					▬	▬	▬						
Yorkshire Fog						▬	▬	▬	▬				
Ryegrass					▬	▬	▬						
Broom					▬	▬	▬						
Fescue					▬	▬							
Timothy							▬						

- Foxtail – pollinates April to June. Foxtail likes to live in damp meadows and pastures. It has a wide distribution throughout Britain.
- Meadowgrass – pollinates May to July. Meadowgrass likes to grow in meadows and on dunes. It grows throughout Britain.
- Ryegrass – pollinates twice, with a major yield from May to July and a lesser yield in August. Ryegrass likes to grow on waste ground but is widely cultivated agriculturally for fodder. It grows well as a lawn and is used in gardens, playing fields and road verges. This is a highly allergenic grass, and consequently a major cause of hayfever.
- Timothy – pollinates in July. Timothy likes to grow in meadows though it is often sown for grass and hay. It has a wide distribution in the southern parts of Britain.
- Vernal – pollinates April to June. As its name (vernal = relating to spring) suggests, it flowers in the spring. Vernal does not have any special preferences for growing sites and tolerates all types of soil. It is distributed throughout Britain.
- Yorkshire Fog – pollinates early June to September. Yorkshire Fog likes fields, woods and waste ground. It grows throughout Britain.

Generally speaking, the protein content of the many different species of grass is surprisingly similar. This means that patients with grass hayfever tend to be challenged with similar proteins whatever the species of grass. This probably explains why grass hayfever is so common. The other big problem is that most of the grasses that cause hayfever are cultivated varieties, meaning that their pollens are present at high levels in areas where people live.

CEREALS AND HAYFEVER

Cereals are special types of grass that are cultivated as food. They tend to cause hayfever problems only in those who live or work near fields of the crop. It is important to realize that cereal pollen hayfever is not the same thing as a reaction to the wheat grain. The wheat grain is, in fact, the ripened seed and contains different proteins from the pollen.

Some people who believe that they suffer from cereal hayfever are in fact reacting to parasitic fungi growing on the surface of the crop. Hayfever-like symptoms caused by fungi are most common at harvest time, when the agitation of the crop causes fungal spores to be thrown into the air.

There are five cereals commonly cultivated in Britain which are as follows.

- Barley – pollinates June and July. Barley is grown in many parts of England and Wales and selected parts of Scotland.
- Maize – pollinates in June and August. Maize is happier growing in warmer climates and is usually cultivated only in southern and eastern England.
- Oats – pollinates July to September. Oats are grown throughout the British Isles, although less commonly in Wales and Ireland.
- Rye – pollinates June to September. Rye is widely grown throughout Britain. The crop rye is related to ryegrass, and consequently, there is a strong cross reactivity.
- Wheat – pollinates June to September. Wheat is grown in low lying areas of Britain.

HOW CAN I REDUCE MY EXPOSURE TO GRASS POLLENS?

The following measures will help to reduce your exposure to grass pollens. Try to follow as many of them as you can. Each suggestion on its own will not cure your hayfever, but when all the measures are combined, the total effect is much greater. Try to avoid going out on warm sunny days during the hayfever season. The pollen count is the highest in the midmorning and late afternoon/evening.

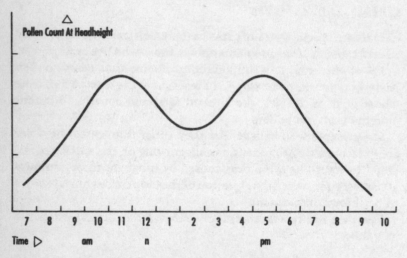

Figure 3.1: Variation of pollen during the day (not to scale)

Pollen is released in large amounts only on warm, sunny days when it is most likely to reach its target. The pollen accumulates at head height in the midmorning before convection currents caused by the heat of the day lift pollen grains up to thousands of feet. In late afternoon and evening the pollen grains that have been taken aloft descend, making the pollen count at head height rise. Cities are hotter than rural areas and, consequently, in cities pollen counts remain high well into the evening. In contrast, in the country the pollen counts drop much earlier. Rain, especially fine rain, usually causes a dramatic drop in the pollen count.

The typical size of grass pollens varies. The size of the grass pollens most likely to cause hayfever range from 20 to 25 microns (1 micron = 1/1000 of a millimetre). Other common grass pollens are 30 to 40 microns.

- Sleep with your bedroom windows closed. Pollens can't penetrate glass.
- Use an air filter to reduce circulating pollen in the rooms you live and work in. An efficient air filter can greatly reduce the pollen level.
- When you are travelling by car or train keep windows closed. When you travel at high speed along the motorway, you are effectively concentrating grains of pollen, and it creates an effect similar to standing in the middle of a field of waving grass.
- Stay in the town and avoid indoor pollinating plants. This is one of the few occasions when air-conditioning may help your health, since it reduces the indoor pollen level to about 1/50th of that outdoors.
- Stay away from fields, parks and gardens and do not cut the grass. Wear dark glasses to keep the pollen away from your eyes.
- Be aware that rain during the pollen season reduces the pollen count, rain before the pollen season increases the pollen count.
- Holiday at the seaside where the pollen count is usually low. This is because the sun heats the land faster than the sea. This causes inland convection currents which usually ensure an onshore wind. Also, because there are no fields of grass out at sea to act as a source of pollen, the air at the seaside is usually pollen-free. Alternatively, you may decide to take your holiday at a place where the grass is not in season: e.g. in June and July go to the southern hemisphere, where it is winter and there is very little pollen. Or go to hilly and mountainous areas with a turbulent airflow. Alpine areas are usually much better than plains.

'RAPESEED FLU'

There is a particularly irritant form of hayfever caused by oil seed rape, a plant with a very bright yellow flower, which pollinates twice between mid-April and early June. This plant is actually insect-pollinated, but is able to produce a severe form of hayfever, resembling influenza, in people living near fields of it. 'Rapeseed flu' is becoming more common because the area under cultivation for oil and animal feed has risen dramatically in the past ten years, probably due to the European Community farming subsidies. There are several theories as to the cause of the oil seed rape 'flu'. These include the suggestion that the problem occurs because of aromatic substances that are given off by the plant. However, it is likely that some cases of 'rapeseed flu' are, in fact, due to poisoning by pesticides and other chemicals applied to the plant throughout the growing cycle.

HOW IS THE POLLEN COUNT MEASURED?

The pollen count is the number of pollen grains per cubic metre. It is measured using a machine that sucks ten litres of air per minute past over a sticky glass plate held behind the sampling nozzle. The machine samples 14.4 cubic metres in 24 hours. The mean pollen concentration is worked out by using a microscope to count the number of grains deposited on the sticky glass plate, from which the number of pollen grains per cubic metre can be calculated.

In the UK in June and July, there are many ways of finding out the pollen count. It is given on TV and radio in the morning, and there are also telephone numbers which give you information about weather and levels of air pollution.

4

Late Season Hayfever and Weed and Flower Pollens

'A rose by any other name ... '

Technically speaking, a weed is any plant growing in a place where it's not supposed to be – like a rose in a cornfield. More pragmatically, weeds are non-cultivated wind-pollinated flowering plants. In fact, weeds are often one of the most common but under-recognized causes of hayfever. In the USA, Ragweed is the major culprit of hayfever symptoms which occur in the late summer and early autumn.

There are three reasons why weeds cause such a major hayfever problem.

- Widespread distribution of weed species
  Weeds are able to grow almost anywhere. They are to be found growing both on cultivated farmland, and on any available waste ground right in the heart of densely populated cities.
- Massive pollen output easily carried by wind
  Many weeds produce a massive amount of pollen. Some individual weed plants release a staggering 1 million grains of pollen per day. Also, these weed pollen grains tend to be relatively small (16 to 25 microns in diameter: 1 micron = 1/1000 millimetre) and in still air take between 4 and 2 minutes respectively to fall from head height. In turbulent air the weed pollen remains airborne for much longer, and some grains of ragweed pollen have been found 400 miles (640 kilometres) out to sea.
- Protein content of weed pollen
  The protein present in weeds has a strong tendency to cause hayfever.

HOW DO WEEDS SPREAD?

Weeds are known to be tenacious and difficult to get rid of when they have taken hold in a patch of ground. However, their seeds spread to new areas by wind, are eaten and carried by birds and animals, and are included in vegetable cargo which is transported in lorries, trains and ships.

Despite the fact that there are a vast number of weed species in Britain and the USA, there are relatively few that cause hayfever. The common hayfever producing weed families include:

- *Compositae* family
    Ragweed, mugwort, wormwood and dandelion
- Plantain family
    English plantain
- Goosefoot family
    Lamb's quarter, tumbleweed and sugar beet
- *Urticaceae* family
    Nettle, pellitory

Table 4.1 gives details of typical pollination times of weeds and flowers in Britain. For USA pollination times see the Appendix.

- Ragweed – pollinates late summer to early autumn in Britain. Ragweed is rarely found in Britain, but in North America it is the most important cause of hayfever. In the USA this weed is almost solely responsible for all cases of late summer and early autumn hayfever. The giant ragweed and common (short) ragweed give the biggest problem.
- Mugwort (Artemisia) – pollinates July to September in Britain. Mugwort likes to grow in a wide variety of habitats including waste ground and hedgerows and near rivers and streams. It has a wide distribution throughout Britain. These produce large amounts of pollen in late summer and early autumn, which is easily carried by the wind.

Table 4.1: Weed and Flower Pollen Chart

Tree	Jan	Feb	Mar	Apr	May	Jun	Jul	Aug	Sep	Oct	Nov	Dec	Comments
Dandelion			▬▬▬▬▬▬▬▬▬▬▬▬▬▬▬▬										
Plantain				▬▬▬▬▬▬▬▬▬▬									
Pellitory						▬▬▬▬▬▬▬▬▬▬▬▬							
Nettle					▬▬▬▬▬▬								
Mugwort						▬▬▬▬▬▬▬▬							
Ragweed							▬▬▬▬▬▬						
Chrysan-themum+ Marguerite						▬▬▬▬▬							
Golden Rod						▬▬▬▬							
Dahlia							▬▬▬▬▬						
Aster						▬▬▬							

- Dandelion - pollinates March to October. Dandelion likes to grow in a very wide variety of habitats including meadows, lawns and waste grounds.
- Plantain - pollinates April to August. Plantain likes to grow amongst grass on acid and neutral, moist sandy or loamy soils. It is found in lawns as well as pastures and meadows. It produces large amounts of pollen in the summer and early autumn, which is easily carried by the wind. It has a wide distribution throughout Britain and the rest of the world.
- The Goosefoot family - pollinates in the late summer. These grow in dry, sandy areas with a low nitrogen content. Although each plant produces a relatively small amount of pollen, because there are such a large number of plants the net result is a high pollen count.
- Nettle - pollinates June to August. Nettle likes to grow in a very wide variety of habitat including hedgerows, woods and grassy places but especially in damp places where there is litter, rubble or near buildings. It has a wide distribution throughout Britain.
- Pellitory - pollinates June to October. Pellitory likes to grow in

hedges and cracks in rocks and decaying buildings. It grows in England, Wales and Ireland.

FLOWERS

Flowers, especially insect pollinated flowers, are rarely a cause of hayfever because they have large sticky pollen grains which are unable to travel far on the wind. Flowers may cause a problem to those who grow them in greenhouses or work in florists' shops. The following flowers are thought to cause problems in some people:

- Aster – pollinates August to September. Aster grows throughout Britain.
- Chrysanthemum – pollinates June to August. This flower is grown for commercial purposes and by enthusiasts.
- Marguerite – pollinates June to August. The Marguerite has a wide distribution throughout Britain, especially on grassland.
- Golden Rod – pollinates June to September. Golden Rod grows naturally in dry areas including woods, grasslands, hedges and cliffs, and is also cultivated. The pollen of the Golden Rod is the flower protein most likely to cause an allergic problem.
- Dahlia – pollinates August to October. Dahlia are widely cultivated throughout Britain.
- Wallflower – pollinates April to July. Wallflowers are often cultivated commercially.

5

'Winter Hayfever' and Fungal Spores

The surprising thing about fungi is not that they cause hayfever-like symptoms but rather, in damp places, that everybody in the area isn't constantly suffering from them. Fungal spores are very small (circa 5 microns: 1 micron = 1/1000 mm) and in wet conditions are produced in astronomically large numbers. It is common for the fungal spore concentration to be 1,000–10,000 per cubic metre in wet places, and in damp enclosed places where vegetable matter is shaken (e.g. moving waterlogged straw in a barn) the level can reach millions per cubic metre.

The saving grace of fungi is that the threshold for appearance of symptoms is usually several thousand spores per cubic metre and, in cold dry winter months, typical fungal spore counts are as low as 1–5 spores per cubic metre.

The very small size of most of the spores guarantees that each individual fungal particle remains suspended for a long time, taking approximately 50 minutes to drop from head height in still air. In slightly turbulent air, the spores remain aloft practically indefinitely. When you compare the mere 200 pollen grains per cubic metre present at the height of the hayfever season with the 1,000 to 10,000 fungal spores per cubic metre to be found in wet places, it is easy to see why fungi are potentially such a major problem to susceptible individuals.

Some patients find that they suffer from hayfever-like symptoms all the year round. This is a condition called *perennial rhinitis*. If the condition is especially bad in places where it is damp and/or in the months of August to October, then a fungal cause for the hayfever-like symptoms must be suspected.

Unlike plants that release pollen only in the flowering season, many fungi constantly release a background level of spores throughout the year. However, like flowering plants, each species of fungi has a time when its sporing activity is highest. If you find that you get hayfever-like symptoms every year during one specific period which is outside the grass hayfever season, then you must suspect a fungal allergy.

IMPORTANT FUNGAL CAUSES OF HAYFEVER-LIKE SYMPTOMS

Outdoor Problems: the following two moulds are the most common causes of outdoor fungal hayfever-like symptoms. Their growth is related to the presence primarily of water, but also of rotting vegetable matter, which is their food source. Their numbers drop dramatically when the first frosts appear.

- Alternaria sporulates in the late summer when the weather is warm and dry. Alternaria is often released into the air near crops like wheat and potato at harvest time when the crop is shaken. It is also present in house dust. Alternaria is unusual in having very large teardrop-shaped spores, 12×33 microns in size. However, it is still one of the commonest causes of fungal perennial rhinitis (hayfever-like symptoms).
- Cladosporium (Hormodendron). Peak sporulation is in July and August, especially during hot dry periods. The spore is teardrop-shaped and is 4×16 microns in size. This fungus mimics the hayfever caused by grasses and weeds. Cladosporium is one of the most important causes of fungal-induced rhinitis and asthma. This is probably related to the exceptionally high level of fungal spores to be found in the air. Quite commonly the concentration of Cladosporium spores is as high as 1,000–10,000 per cubic metre.

Indoor Problems: the following three moulds are the most common cause of indoor fungal hayfever-like symptoms. They grow throughout the year and live on rotting food like bread and overripe fruit, in basements, garden sheds, kitchens and bathrooms and on moist bedding.

- Aspergillus sporulates throughout the year. This grows on rotten grasses and is found in compost heaps and wet straw. It is most common during the winter months because of the large amount of rotting vegetation. In houses it grows very widely in all the places listed above. Its selective advantage over other fungi seems to be that it is able to live with a relatively low moisture content.
- Mucor/Rhizopus – these related moulds sporulate all year round. They live on overripe food and are found in house dust. They are an important source of perennial rhinitis.
- Penicillium sporulates throughout the year. It appears as a blue/green mould growing on decaying fruits and occurring in house dust; also as the black marks found on damp wallpaper and window ledges and other damp surfaces.

OTHER FUNGAL CAUSES OF HAYFEVER-LIKE SYMPTOMS

- Botrytis sporulates in late summer and autumn. This is a mould that lives on the surface of grain and also on strawberries, cucumbers and potatoes.
- Candida albicans sporulates throughout the year. It is a white mould which in the body can cause thrush, a very wide variety of symptoms due to Candida overgrowth in the bowel and athlete's foot. It likes a warm, wet environment, and is encouraged to grow by antibiotics, steroids, the oral contraceptive pill and pregnancy.
- Chaetomium sporulates all the year round. It grows on wet straw, fibres and dung, but is rare in Britain.
- Curvularia sporulates June till September. It lives on cereals and is sometimes found in house dust.

- Fusarium sporulates throughout the year. It is a white or colourless mould which grows on a wide variety of fruit and vegetables including potatoes, cabbage, tomato, cereal, bananas and cotton.
- Helminthosporium sporulates in August and September. It grows on cereals and rotting vegetable matter.
- Micropolyspora sporulates throughout the year, especially in late autumn and winter. It lives on damp hay, causing heat production and is one of the causes of 'Farmer's Lung'.
- Neurospora sporulates all round the year. It is often found in bakeries as a red bread mould.
- Phoma sporulates particularly in the early autumn. It is a black coloured fungus that grows on beet and citrus fruits, and rotting vegetation; an important cause of fungal problems.
- Pullularia sporulates in the summer. Grows on fruit and vegetables and painted surfaces that get persistently wet.
- Sporobolomyces sporulates during damp, warm conditions. Lives in damp places near trees and rivers.
- Surpula (dry rot) sporulates throughout the year. Grows on moist, poorly ventilated wood in old buildings. May cause rhinitis and asthma. Many of the human health problems associated with this fungus are in fact a result of poisoning with the pesticides used to treat the dry rot. Such treatment causes problems to people working and sleeping near to such infested wood up to 5 years after treatment. The best cure for dry rot is to replace the wood and ensure that the replaced timber is no longer wet.
- Trichophyton sporulates throughout the year. Found in the soil and causes the foot infection tinea pedis.
- Ustilago sporulates especially in July. A dry powdery deposit (smut) on grain, may cause summer symptoms.

By far the most important clue that should lead you to suspect that you may have a fungal problem is the presence of water. This may be present as visible liquid or just as damp, condensation or humidity. Fungi need lots of water to grow and reproduce and are attracted anywhere that moisture is freely available. Indoors this means bathrooms and showers, under sinks with leaky plumbing, in basements and near damp spots caused by rising damp, leaking roofs and any other source of water. Outdoors, this means in poorly drained, shaded spots, especially if there is a plentiful supply of rotting vegetation which acts as an excellent food supply. The characteristic musty smell should give you a vital clue as to the presence of fungi, especially if you start sneezing within a couple of minutes of being in such places.

If you suspect that you have a fungal allergy, you can confirm your suspicion by the use of the prick test and the RAST test (see page 32).

AREAS WHERE FUNGI ARE MOST LIKELY TO BE FOUND

The level of rainfall and relative humidity in different climates greatly affect fungal growth. In northern latitudes such as Britain, the northern states of the USA and Scandinavia, where the relative humidity is generally lower, between 4 and 10 per cent of patients suffering from atopy (see page 32) react to the common fungi. However, in latitudes closer to the equator, where the humidity level is generally higher, between 20 and 30 per cent of patients with atopic problems react to fungi.

Buildings and Fungi

Although fungi are most likely to occur in dusty, humid places, enough spores can accumulate in an apparently clean dry building to cause problems. Far more importantly, air-conditioning systems, especially the part responsible for humidifying the air, may act as a focus for the multiplication of these spores. There is even a condition described as 'humidifier fever', which occurs especially after a weekend or holiday break, which is due to the occupants of the building being sprayed with large numbers of fungal spores, and also bacteria, through the air ducts. Those patients who already have allergies, with a compromised immune system, or who suffer from Candida are especially likely to be affected by this problem.

WHEN ARE FUNGI MOST LIKELY TO SPORULATE?

Fungi grow all the year round, but the fungal spore count is usually at its peak from August to October. As well as seasonal variation there is hour to hour and day to day variation. Once again the key to the fungal spore count is water. Spore counts are highest in the early morning, when the dew is about, and on days when it has been raining. If you sneeze after thunderstorms, it is likely that your hayfever-like symptoms are caused by fungi.

COMMON SYMPTOMS OF FUNGAL 'ALLERGY'

As well as causing hayfever-like symptoms fungi can cause symptoms affecting the whole body. The common picture of fungal allergy is a constant flu-like state, which may persist even during brief periods away from the fungal source. Recurrent tiredness is common, especially when there is also a high load of Candida. This may be mistaken for ME. There may also be many mental symptoms including headache, poor memory and concentration, confusion, irritability, mood swings and depression.

WHICH FACTORS ARE LIKELY TO MAKE AN INDIVIDUAL MORE SUSCEPTIBLE TO FUNGAL PROBLEMS?

Any factor that increases the load of neotoxins (20th-century poisons: see chapter 8) increases the risk of a fungal problem, but the common predisposing factors include long-term use of antibiotics or steroids, the contraceptive pill, and multiple pregnancies. Also a diet rich in sugar, refined carbohydrates, yeast, cheese, alcohol or vinegar, and finally exposure to damp and moulds.

6

'All Year Round Hayfever': House Dust Mite and Animals

If you suffer hayfever-like symptoms all the year round **inside your home**, then the most likely cause is the house dust mite, followed by pets and animals. In dry houses, moulds and pollen are usually a relatively unimportant cause of such symptoms.

The hayfever-like reaction to animal proteins is a common problem, especially amongst atopic patients who also suffer from eczema or asthma. But the good news is that these symptoms can be cured completely by avoiding contact with the offending mite or animal and its proteins.

The best way to identify the underlying cause of indoor hayfever that persists all the year round is by careful questioning and possibly skin prick or RAST testing. This chapter gives a little more information about the common causes and list the measures can then be taken to reduce exposure.

HOUSE DUST MITE

Houses dust mites are microscopic transparent spider-like creatures (1/3 mm = 300 microns long) that live in almost everybody's home in Britain and the USA. They produce faecal particles of between 1 and 20 microns in diameter which are so small that they remain airborne for a considerable time. The mites are usually at their highest level in the bedroom and live primarily in mattresses but also in upholstery, carpets and curtains.

House dust mites feed on human skin scales, and an adult person loses ½ to 1 g of scales per day, much of which ends up in their bed. Consequently, the average mattress which has been used for some time contains 10,000 to 100,000 house dust mites. House dust mites prefer warm moist places. As a rule of thumb, the greater the amount of moisture in the air, the higher the house dust mite level in beds, carpets, sofas and curtains. High levels of indoor moisture are encouraged by modern construction methods emphasizing small rooms, low ventilation with high insulation, and humidity. House dust mites can't cope with dry conditions, sunlight and boil washes (hotter than 58°C).

Measures to reduce the house dust mite level include:

- Living in a house that is dry and sited away from open water and underground streams;
- Avoiding open fires that burn coal, gas and paraffin, which produce a lot of water vapour and so increase humidity;
- Ensuring good ventilation, especially in the bedroom, to avoid the build-up of humidity;
- Buying a new mattress, preferably without buttons, and have it on a wooden frame rather than a divan;
- Covering the mattress with a special microporous mattress cover. This cover allows the mattress to 'breathe' and moisture to pass in and out, but prevents skin scales from entering the mattress and the house dust mites and their faeces from leaving the mattress. This single measure can be spectacularly successful. The alternative measure of using a waterproof plastic sheet is less successful and may even encourage growth of fungi in the mattress which is unable to 'breathe'.
- Remove pillows and eiderdowns filled with feathers, since the house dust mite may live on the feathers. Replace them with ones filled with natural fibres - like cellular cotton blankets. Use cotton blankets on your bed.
- If you sleep in a bunk bed, take the upper bed. This stops mites falling onto you.

The other measures to reduce house dust mites are all down to housework, which ideally should be carried out by someone who is not allergic to the house dust mite.

- Vacuum all around the bed, mattress and carpets around the bed each week. Infants are most likely to be sensitive by breathing in house dust mites from carpets, since the house dust mites are unable to survive on their plastic mattress covers. Also, vacuum all other furniture and in crevices. Use a cylinder vacuum cleaner with a disposable paper dust bag or, even better, a vacuum cleaner with a water-filled trap to filter the exhaust air. Upright vacuum cleaners with cloth bags often merely throw the house dust mite into the atmosphere and are counter-productive. Don't forget to vacuum all beds in the room. Vacuuming removes the house dust mite but it does not remove any sticky eggs, which remain in the mattress.
- Wash all sheets, blankets, duvet and pillow cases on the bed. Use a boil wash, as the house dust mite eggs are heat resistant.
- Be sure to remove soft, furry toys taken to bed and give them a boil wash. They sometimes act as a massive reservoir of the house dust mite.
- Damp dust all surfaces in the room, e.g. window ledges, tops of furniture, pelmets. Don't use a dry brush, since it propels house dust mites into the atmosphere.
- Air your mattress at least once a month. The house dust mite dislikes sunlight and dry air. If the weather is cold but dry, then air your mattress outside, since the intense cold kills the house dust mite. House dust mites cannot live in dry, cold conditions or at higher altitudes, such as are found in the alpine areas.
- Do *not* use insecticides to kill the house dust mite. It is often ineffective and the insecticide may cause you to suffer a chemical sensitivity. One drastic but effective way to reduce house dust mites is to get a contractor to douse your mattress with liquid nitrogen. This is a very effective way to greatly reduce the mite population.
- Use air filtration equipment. This greatly reduces the number of circulating particles in the air with consequent improvement. Ionizers are also helpful in reducing the number of circulating particles by giving them a negative charge, which attracts them to surfaces in the room which are usually positively charged.

PETS AND ANIMALS

After the house dust mites, the second biggest culprit causing hayfever-like symptoms *indoors* are pets. Cats cause the biggest problem, followed by dogs and then the list runs to other pets, like gerbils, guinea pigs, hamsters, mice, rabbits and rats. The protein causing the hayfever-like symptoms may be the hair, skin scales (dander), saliva or urine.

Avoidance of animal protein is more difficult than it sounds. Even finding another home for the animal may not be an immediate answer. After a pet leaves your house, it may take up to 2 years to get rid of the last traces of its occupation. This explains why hayfever-like symptoms sometimes persist. Furthermore, direct contact with the pet is not necessary, since the animal proteins dry to form small particles which easily become and remain airborne.

Cats

Cats are the commonest cause of pet-induced hayfever-like symptoms. The cat protein causing the biggest problem is the one found in saliva, with which the animal coats its fur when grooming. The cat saliva protein forms very small particles (less than 2.5 microns: 1 micron = 1/1000 millimetre). These tiny particles easily become airborne, explaining how cat-induced hayfever can occur without direct contact with the animal. In addition, these cat saliva protein particles are resistant to indoor weathering, and persist unchanged for months in uncleaned rooms.

Dogs

Dogs produce hayfever-like symptoms because of proteins in skin scales (dander), hair, urine, faeces, saliva and even blood. Some patients believe they react to long-haired breeds but not to the short-haired ones, however, the problem is more likely to be related to the amount of skin scales shed, rather than the length of hair.

Other Animals

Guinea pigs, hamsters and rabbits and are usually kept outside and consequently because of the greatly increased ventilation and lower concentration of protein in the air are less of a problem. Other pets which are kept indoors like gerbils, mice and rats may be troublesome, especially if allowed in the bedroom and/or if their cages are not cleaned regularly.

Laboratory Animals

Laboratory animals such as rats, mice, guinea pigs and rabbits are often kept in poorly ventilated cages. At least 1 in 10 laboratory workers becomes allergic to these animals due to repeated exposure and suffers hayfever-like symptoms. Although the problem can be caused by the animal hair or skin scales, a more frequent cause is the proteins from the urine and/or faeces, which dry on the cage floor and become airborne. A similar problem can also occur in sheds used to rear battery hens.

Feathers

Feathers either come from caged birds and/or pigeon lofts/dovecots or else are also found in pillows, cushions, quilts and eiderdowns. It is very important that both sources should all be avoided by people with a feather allergy. However, there are some patients who believe that they have a feather allergy when in fact the real problem is one with house dust mites living on the feathers.

Horses

Allergic reaction to horses is common amongst those who are in frequent contact with horses and horse manure. The likely situations for problems include:

stable/racecourse exposure
agricultural exposure
amateur riders.

Some sensitive patients may react to the horse hair used to stuff furniture and mattresses.

TREATING PET-INDUCED HAYFEVER

By far the best way to cope with pet-induced hayfever is to get rid of the animal. In many cases, this is not a realistic option but the following measures often prove helpful:

- Don't allow pets in your bedroom. Let them live, sleep and be groomed in parts of the house that you can avoid;
- Keep pets in an area that can be easily washed (e.g. linoleum or vinyl floors), since this will prevent build-up of animal hairs;
- Avoid situations and occupations where you will come into contact with animals; e.g. pet owners and their houses, zoos, circuses, farmers and vets;
- Use air filtration equipment. This greatly reduces the number of circulating particles in the air with consequent improvement. Ionizers are also helpful in reducing the number of circulating particles by giving them a negative charge, which attracts them to surfaces which are usually positively charged.
- Don't buy pets in future and, after they have gone, replace carpets and floor coverings and thoroughly clean upholstery.

OTHER CAUSES OF HAYFEVER-LIKE SYMPTOMS

There are other lesser appreciated causes of hayfever-like symptoms, including exposure to cockroaches and their faeces. This is a particular problem in large, old, multiple-occupier buildings and institutions where there is a poor standard of hygiene.

TESTING AND AVOIDING SENSITIZATION

Once again the prick test and the RAST test are the most helpful ways of discovering which animal protein you are reacting to (see page 32).

The human body is most likely to become sensitized to an allergy-producing protein (e.g. house dust mite, cat/dog, fungi, pollen) if exposed between 3 and 6 months after birth. This phenomenon was first demonstrated with Silver Birch pollen in Scandinavia. It was found that children born in September were more likely to develop Silver Birch hayfever because the pollen levels were highest from January to March when babies were 3–6 months old.

A similar vulnerability to sensitization occurs with house dust mites, pets and feathers. There is an 'allergy window' between 3 and 6 months, when the baby's immune system is not yet fully competent, and the maternal antibodies given to the baby before birth start to drop to low levels. Consequently it is particularly important that babies are not exposed to high levels of mite, pet and bird proteins between 3 and 6 months.

7

Other Conditions that Mimic Hayfever

Few diseases are completely clear-cut and straightforward. Hayfever is no exception to this general rule. So far this book has dealt with classical hayfever caused by an immunological reaction between pollen, IgE antibodies and mast cells. However, there are at least three conditions that are able to mimic hayfever symptoms but do not involve the IgE/Mast cell reaction. These three conditions, which are compared in table 7.1, are:

- vasomotor rhinitis – caused by the stimulation of nerves, making the nose more sensitive to environmental factors and pollution
- drug-induced rhinitis – caused by a wide variety of prescribed and over-the-counter drugs
- non-specific rhinitis – caused by a very wide variety of factors including foods and chemicals.

The mechanisms which cause these non-IgE/mast cell allergic reactions will be explained in chapter 8, but it is useful to describe the symptoms here.

VASOMOTOR RHINITIS

This is a condition whose cause is a non-IgE/mast cell reaction. However, the lining of the nose becomes excessively sensitive to irritants like pollution, smoke, alcohol, temperature change and emotion. There is often an element of vasomotor rhinitis in

Table 7.1: The difference between IgE/mast cell hayfever and other forms of rhinitis

	IgE/mast cell hayfever	Vasomotor Rhinitis	Drug-induced Rhinitis	Non-specific Rhinitis
Age of onset	Child or adult	Adult	Adult	Adult
Delay between exposure and symptom	Minutes	Minutes	7-10 days	Variable
Sneezing/ itching	Severe	Absent	Absent	Mild
Runny nose	Moderate	Moderate	Severe	Moderate
Skin prick reaction	Marked	Absent	Absent	Absent
Development nasal polyp	Unlikely	Very unlikely	Likely	Likely

classical hayfever and it can be difficult to distinguish between the two conditions.

DRUG-INDUCED RHINITIS

Some drugs may induce hayfever-like symptoms in a susceptible patient. Table 7.1 will help you distinguish between drug-induced rhinitis and other forms. The drug-induced rhinitis may be caused by very tiny amounts of a very wide variety of drugs but, fortunately, when the medication is discontinued, symptoms usually disappear rapidly.

Drug-induced rhinitis is most likely to occur in individuals with a defective detoxification system who are already ill. The typical sufferer is over 55, female and with previous history of drug reactions such as rashes, dizziness and nausea, and also a family history of allergy. The drugs that sometimes cause reactions include:

- Anaesthetics
- Antiarthritic drugs, especially aspirin and related drugs
- Antibiotics – penicillin, sulphonamides, nitrofurans and anti-TB drugs
- Antiepileptic drugs
- Antifungals
- Antigout medication
- Antimalarials
- Anti-hyperthyroid drugs
- Blood pressure medication
- Heart medication to stop palpitations
- Heavy metals – gold
- Muscle relaxants
- Organ extracts – insulin, ACTH
- Sleeping tablets
- Tranquillizers
- Vaccines and antisera
- X-ray contrast media containing iodine

NON-SPECIFIC RHINITIS

This is a non-IgE/mast cell allergic condition. It may be caused by a very wide variety of substances including foods, chemicals such as formaldehyde, pesticides, solvents, paints and glues and is basically a condition known as chemical sensitivity. Non-specific rhinitis or chemical sensitivity is a major contribution to the explosion in the incidence of hayfever. This large topic is dealt with in greater depth in chapter 11.

HOW DO THESE CONDITIONS MIMIC HAYFEVER?

The basic reason why these alternative causes of 'hayfever' are able to mimic the classical symptoms is that each makes the mast cell release histamine directly. Although the histamine is not released via the IgE/mast cell route, it has a similar effect on the eyes and nose. Figure 7.1 illustrates some of the alternative ways that histamine may be released.

Figure 7.1: Factors able to release histamine from mast cells

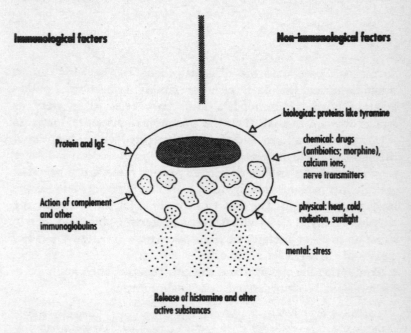

Immunological factors   Non-immunological factors

Protein and IgE

Action of complement
and other
immunoglobulins

biological: proteins like tyramine

chemical: drugs
(antibiotics; morphine),
calcium ions,
nerve transmitters

physical: heat, cold,
radiation, sunlight

mental: stress

Release of histamine and other
active substances

8

Hayfever and the Total Load Concept

$$2 + 2 = 5$$

So far you have read the classical theory of hayfever; unfortunately, in real life, hayfever is not simply a question of pollen reacting with IgE antibodies and mast cells. If it were as straightforward as that, then the symptoms suffered by patients would be more uniform, and more easily treated with conventional medicines. Due to the high levels of pollution of air, food and water now so common in the developed world, there are now other allergic mechanisms which are at least partly responsible for the hayfever symptoms. The function of this chapter is to see the existing theory of classical hayfever as a starting point and then to move on to other allergic mechanisms, which are often the major causes of the hayfever symptoms.

Combining the classical and the new theories, the likelihood of hayfever can be summarized in a single formula:

$$\frac{\text{Likelihood of}}{\text{hayfever}} = \frac{\text{Pollen}}{\text{challenge}} \times \frac{\text{Proximity}}{\text{to source}} \times \frac{\text{Time}}{\text{exposed}} \times \frac{\text{Competence of}}{\text{immune system}}$$

These individual concepts have been dealt with in previous chapters and the first formula is of fundamental importance in Environmental Medicine.

WHAT ARE THE OTHER ALLERGIC MECHANISMS RESPONSIBLE FOR HAYFEVER?

So far in examining hayfever, we have looked at only one type of allergic reaction (type I hypersensitivity), in which a foreign protein

Figure 8.1

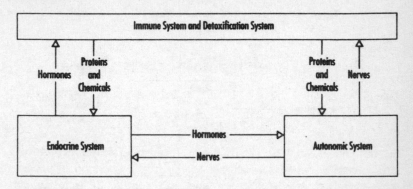

(pollen) reacts with a pollen-specific antibody (IgE), releasing histamine from the mast cell. However, this in an excessively narrow definition of allergy. The original definition used by Clemens von Pirquet in 1906 was much broader and included *any* altered reaction (Greek: *allos* - other; *ergon* - work or reaction).

Although immunologists have tried to confuse the situation by introducing their narrow definition off allergy, the true definition is any abnormal reaction to a 'foreign' substance (a neotoxin or 20th-century poison - see below for definition). This reaction may occur at any time after the first exposure when the 'foreign' substance enters the body through the mouth (eating or drinking), lungs (inhaled), or skin (contact). The unpleasant reaction is produced by the immune system and a failure of the detoxification system. The immune system is composed of white cells and antibodies which both circulate in the blood. The detoxification system is composed of enzymes which occur in every cell of the body, but especially in the liver. The immune system is controlled by hormones like adrenaline and hydrocortisone, and these have an important effect on the autonomic nervous system which works automatically and controls essential functions like breathing, heart rate, and function of bowels and bladder. The enzymes of the

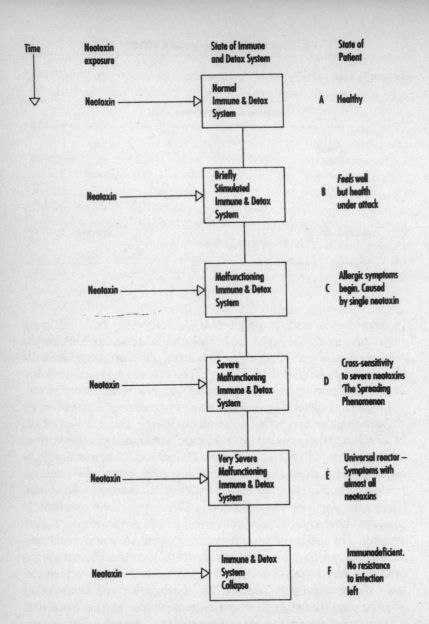

Figure 8.2: Progression of allergy and state of Immune and Detoxification System after continued exposure to neotoxin

detoxification system break down foreign substances that enter the body, and excrete them either through the liver (faeces), kidneys (urine), skin (sweat) or sexual secretions.

The interrelation of the immune, detoxification, endocrine and autonomic systems is shown in figure 8.1.

The normal function of the immune system is to inspect all substances entering the body and decide whether they are harmless (e.g. organic foods), or harmful (e.g. bacteria, viruses, fungi and parasites). People with allergies have a defective immune system that wrongly identifies harmless molecules as harmful intruders, and/or a defective detoxification system that is unable to get rid of the offending substances. It also overreacts to chemicals and pollutants (neotoxins) giving rise to a wide variety of poorly defined symptoms which may affect any of the body systems - often several systems simultaneously (e.g. headache, arthritis, colitis). See figure 8.2.

The presence of a foreign substance or neotoxin briefly causes a heightened sensitivity which stimulates the immune system and detoxification system to work harder. The immune system works harder by producing antibodies, many sorts of proteins and extra white cells; the detoxification system works harder by producing more enzymes. This process of induction of enzymes is termed *adaption* (A). (B) is then replaced by (C) in which malfunctioning immune and detoxification systems give allergic symptoms to a single neotoxin (e.g. formaldehyde). If neotoxin exposure continues (D), the immune and detoxification systems become much less discriminating and a 'spreading phenomenon' occurs in which there is a cross-sensitivity to many chemicals and substances. The immune and detoxification systems react to any neotoxin that has a chemical similarity to the initial one. If exposure continues (E) - rarely - the immune and detoxification systems begin to respond adversely to almost everything (e.g. most foods, and chemicals), and the person becomes a 'universal reactor'. Very occasionally, if exposure to the neotoxin continues, the immune and detoxification systems go into a state of collapse (F) and the patient has little or no resistance left to any infection.

WHAT CAUSES ALLERGIES?

Allergies are caused by neotoxins, which are poisons of the 20th century.

Definition: A neotoxin is a very broad term used to describe any sort of harmful agent which may cause an environmentally induced illness, often called an 'allergy', in a susceptible individual. The sources of allergies are:

* Biological
  Food and drink, bacterial, viral and fungal infections, and parasites, plant and animal proteins.
* Chemical
  A vast range including petrochemicals, pesticides, toxic metals.
* Physical
  Electromagnetic radiation (e.g. radio, microwaves, X rays, cosmic rays), sound and vibration, geopathic stress.
* Mental
  Stress.

The term allergy is a very loose one, but the mechanism occurring in most allergies is that neotoxins cause production of excess *free radicals* within cells. Free radicals are atoms or molecules with a positive or negative charge due to one or more unpaired outer electrons, e.g. hydrogen atom, molecular oxygen and metals such as iron or copper. Free radicals are essential for cells to release energy and are only destructive when they become present in excess numbers. They are removed by the detoxification system i.e. antioxidant enzymes such as superoxide dismutase and antioxidant vitamins (C, E and beta-carotene).

Biological, chemical, physical and mental neotoxins are all able to produce excess free radicals which then overwhelm the cell's antioxidant capacity. If free radicals are not removed then they may start a chain reaction causing a cascade of further toxic products. The free radicals can cause major damage to cells by:

- attacking the fats in cell membranes, causing them to become more permeable and let in substances that are usually kept out;
- attacking proteins including enzymes and DNA (genetic material), stopping them from working properly;
- altering glucose metabolism so that toxic substances are produced.

Allergies develop when free radicals are produced faster than the detoxification system's ability to remove them. The accumulated free radicals (the *total load of neotoxins*) cause the tissue damage and breakdown in function that is called allergy.

THE INCREASING INCIDENCE OF ALLERGIES

Most allergies are between two and ten times more common than they were 40 years ago. There are three basic reasons for this massive change.

1. The vastly increased load of chemical neotoxins in air, food and water. Pollution of air, food and water causes neotoxins to build up, or *bioaccumulate*, in the body and when the total load gets above the threshold for illness an allergy occurs.
2. Vastly increased indoor air pollution as a result of modern building methods. Modern buildings are made using materials that give off lots of toxic chemicals, especially formaldehyde, but the buildings are made airtight and the greatly reduced ventilation does not allow these chemicals to escape.
3. Modern production methods yield food that is deficient in essential nutrients such as vitamins, minerals, and essential fatty acids.

HOW DO NEOTOXINS CAUSE ALLERGIES?

Neotoxins (e.g. food additives, pesticides) produce allergies by causing a malfunction of the immune and detoxification systems which then cause secondary damage in other tissues of the body. This damage is initially caused by free radicals followed by inflammation which causes the release of highly reactive substances such as histamine and prostaglandins. The result of histamine is irritation, leakage of fluid from blood vessels and swelling.

There is controversy among scientists as to how allergy damages the immune system. Some of the suggested ways include:

- Toxicity

  This is due to a direct or indirect toxic effect of the neotoxin (e.g. lead, mercury and other heavy metals) on the immune system and detoxification systems. The detoxification system is overwhelmed by a small amount of an excessively toxic substance, or a less toxic substance present at too high a level.

- Irritation

  This is due to release of histamine and other highly reactive substances by the neotoxin (e.g. acids and alkalis).

- Pharmacological

  Many neotoxins (e.g. alcohol, caffeine, nicotine) have a drug-like action on the body. These cause their effects by stimulating 'receptors' on the surface of the cells. These 'receptors' identify specific substances due to the shape of the molecule.

- Immunological reactions

  The immune system produces antibodies which circulate in the blood. These antibodies cause the release of histamine (as in hayfever) and join with foreign proteins to produce immune complexes which can cause activation of the 'complement' system and white cells which then produce tissue damage (e.g. contact dermatitis).

- Non-immunological reactions

  This is a very large category and is the cause of a large proportion of allergic problems, although the precise mechanism is not known.

- Intolerance

  This is caused by enzymes not working properly. Enzymes are

catalysts produced by the body to assist the biochemical conversion of one substance to another. Enzyme malfunctions can be 'fixed' (non-repairable) or 'non-fixed' (repairable with time). See below.

A 'fixed' enzyme defect is caused by a damaged gene inherited from one or other parent. It is unlikely to heal, and the possessor of this gene will have an allergic problem throughout life, e.g. coeliac disease, in which the patient cannot eat gluten which is a protein present in wheat.

A 'non-fixed' enzyme defect occurs because an enzyme is overused and it becomes 'bruised' – e.g. temporary milk allergy often occurs in infants after a bowel infection. If the enzyme system is 'rested' for a short time (two to six months), then it is usually able to repair itself wholly or partly, and the body goes into a state of 'tolerance'. In this state of 'tolerance' it is possible to take occasionally (once a week) the neotoxin that previously gave problem without allergic symptoms.

ALLERGIC ILLNESSES

Hayfever is just one of the wide range of illnesses and symptoms that are caused by allergy – when the total load of neotoxins is too high. These include: arthritis, rheumatism, asthma, bronchitis, wheezing, a 'doped up' feeling, drowsiness, epilepsy, headache, feeling 'high', hyperactivity, irritability, light sensitivity, migraine, muscular weakness, pins and needles, restless legs, sleep disorders, visual, hearing and balance problems, bed wetting, cystitis, frequency of urination, genital itch, infertility, thrush, dermatitis, eczema, addiction, anxiety, depression, panic attacks, phobias, recurrent infections, blocked nose, glue ear, angina, circulation problems, faints, fast pulse, high blood pressure, irregular pulse, abdominal pain, bloating, colic, colitis, constipation, diarrhoea, excessive hunger, irritable bowel syndrome, obesity, excessive thirst, thyroid disease and menstrual problems.

FACTORS AFFECTING THE DEVELOPMENT OF ALLERGY

Heredity
Allergic tendency can be inherited. See p 32.

Age and Sex
Allergic disease is commoner in young infants and children, especially boys, many allergies **apparently** curing themselves by the age of 20 years. Adult women are almost twice as likely to suffer from allergies as men.

Nutrition
This is the single most important factor that influences the development of allergy. Its importance starts before birth when the baby is growing in the mother's womb. If the mother does not smoke or drink alcohol, if she avoids bingeing on the same few foods (by rotating unpolluted organic foods and drinking spring water), and has adequate mineral and vitamin intakes, she greatly reduces the likelihood of allergy in her child. See chapter 14 for more on this topic.

Hormonal State
The immune and detoxification systems are influenced by hormones. The level of hormones varies with time of day (circadian rhythm) and for women, time of the month (menstrual cycle). The time of day when you have greatest susceptibility to illness is 4.00 am. For women the time of the month of greatest susceptibility to illness is the week before their period.

Other Habits
Alcohol, smoking and drugs (prescribed or otherwise) all take their toll on the immune system. Sex with many different partners increases the risk of infection and consequent neotoxin load. Women may have an extra problem in this area, in that semen contains a high doses of 'foreign' proteins and the substance pro-staglandin. Both of these will challenge a woman's immune system.

General State of Health
This influences how much resistance a person has to further challenges.

Total Load of Neotoxins
This is a fundamental concept in Environmental Medicine. The state of your immune system is very strongly influenced by your **total load of neotoxins.** If your food and drink have many additives and/or you are exposed to many chemicals, and/or electromagnetic radiations and have a highly stressed lifestyle, then you are more likely to suffer an allergic problem. *The higher the total load, the greater the risk of allergy.*

Allergic symptoms commence when the total load of neotoxins exceed the threshold of the immune and detoxification systems' ability to cope. The total load, however, varies unpredictably from day to day, as does the body's threshold for suffering symptoms, hence explaining the variability of allergic problems.

WHAT ARE THE COMMON SOURCES OF NEOTOXINS?

The neotoxins that contribute to the total load of neotoxins are listed below.

Biological Neotoxins
These have increased year on year since the Second World War when intensive farming methods started in earnest. Food poisoning (an infection) is now depressingly common and most non-organic meat contains hormones, antibiotics and food additives. Water supplies are treated with chemicals, or pesticides and metals.

Chemicals
One hundred years ago there were approximately 150 chemicals in common use. Now there are 60,000. The consumer society has flooded the world with petrochemical fumes and pesticide residues. In addition, organic chemists have succeeded in

producing chemicals that are much more dangerous because they contain the halogenated carbon-chlorine bond (halocarbon), which the body finds very difficult to detoxify. These halocarbons appear to cause much more damage to the immune system, and sources include PCBs from electrical devices, organochlorine, pesticides, cleaning solvents and CFCs in refrigerators, old aerosols and foam containers used for takeaway foods.

Physical
One hundred years ago there were no household electrical devices, and consequently, very few manmade electric and magnetic fields. In the western world it is now impossible to find a population who do not live in an 'electric smog' created by heating and lighting circuits, but especially emitted from motors and transformers.

Mental
A high level of mental stress is now the expected norm for city dwellers. Mental stress contributes to the total load of neotoxins and makes the body more susceptible to an allergy.

WHAT DECIDES IF I WILL SUFFER FROM A NEOTOXIN?

The factors that decide whether you will suffer from a neotoxin are:

- The total load of neotoxins (biological, chemical, physical and mental)
- Individual susceptibility. This is determined by two factors:
   a) the set of genes you inherit from your parents
   b) general state of health

The inherited portion of your individual susceptibility cannot be changed. However, the acquired portion is dependent on your environment, and you can change it to such an extent that you cancel out most genetic defects. The genes you inherit will decide whether you have any defective enzymes. These defective enzymes can cause disease which may be revealed by environmental challenges.

The dose of neotoxins received by a person can be worked out by using the formula:

$$\text{Dose of neotoxin} = \text{Amount of neotoxin} \times \text{Proximity to source of neotoxin} \times \text{Time exposed to neotoxin}$$

However, the dose is not the same as the biological effect, which can be worked out by using the formula:

$$\text{Biological effect} = \text{Dose of neotoxin} \times \text{Individual suspectibility to neotoxin}$$

and

$$\text{Individual Susceptibility} = \text{Genetic influences} \times \text{Acquired environmental influences}$$

The way to beat allergies is explained more fully in chapter 12 but there are three basic rules:

- Reduce your total load of neotoxins.
- Reduce the neotoxin(s) to which you are particularly susceptible.
- Use sleep, rest, exercise, vitamin and mineral supplements to get yourself back to positive health.

By far the most important factor suggesting that a symptom or disease is caused by an environmental factor is *variations in the severity of indicators of health*. If the severity of a symptom or disease varies from time to time or place to place, then there is a high likelihood that the underlying cause is an environmental factor. This is likely to be the cause with your hayfever. Equally importantly, by reducing the total load of neotoxins on the body to the to the minimum, it is usually possible to remain in peak health for your age, sex and previous life history.

Figure 8.3: Scale of Health

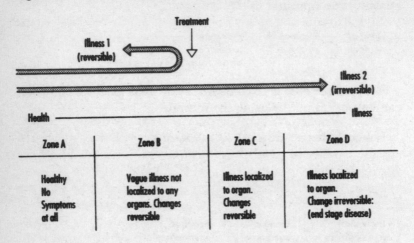

CONVENTIONAL MEDICINE'S WAY OF TREATING ALLERGIES

Conventional medicine treats allergic disease by giving tablets, (antihistamines), and creams, (steroids), that **suppress** the symptoms. This is basically a flawed approach to treatment. The best way to treat allergies is not just to treat the symptom(s) but to remove the cause i.e. the neotoxin.

The symptoms caused by the neotoxin are often the body's attempt to heal itself. For example, diarrhoea is the body's attempt to flush out the offending substance from the bowel. In the same way, in hayfever a runny nose is trying to flush out pollen from the nostrils. To suppress these compensatory mechanisms is merely directing the problem into another system. For example, when topical steroid creams are used to treat eczema the skin eruption disappears but the problem is often transferred to the lungs and there is an increased likelihood of asthma.

A large proportion of patients attending their family doctor are unable to define their problem precisely. They complain of vague symptoms with descriptions of 'feeling off', 'under the weather', 'tired all the time and having no energy'.

To understand the reason for this, it is helpful to look at the several stages that any disease goes through as shown in the Scale of Health in figure 8.3.

Figure 8.3 gives the range of health/illness, from complete health, at the left-hand side of the diagram, to complete illness, at the right-hand side of the diagram. In the first stage of disease (Zone B), the body is exposed to a neotoxin, e.g. a virus, and the illness produced is vague and cannot be localized to any one organ. At this stage the disease is still reversible. If the neotoxin exposure continues the illness becomes localized to a system, e.g. a temporary pain in the joint, but is still reversible (stage C). If no further steps are taken to modify and improve the lifestyle then the illness becomes irreversible, (Zone D), causing permanent illness (e.g. arthritis). The ideal time to act is when the disease is in Zone B or Zone C when the allergy is still reversible and a full recovery is possible (as in illness 1). In comparison, treatment of irreversible disease in Zone D (end-stage disease) is difficult and perfect results cannot normally be obtained (as in illness 2).

WHAT SETS OFF ALLERGIES? (THE TRIGGER EVENT)

Many diseases including allergic ones, often occur following a *trigger event*, such as an accident, bereavement, infection or massive exposure to a neotoxin. Once the illness has started, there is often a permanent change, and the illness continues even if the trigger event is then removed.

The reason that an illness occurs after a trigger event is due to a hidden weakness. This weakness only becomes apparent after an accident, shock, infection or massive exposure to a neotoxin reveals the problem. People who have a hidden weakness to a neotoxin require a relatively small 'push' or trigger event to precipitate their allergic disease. Other people without this hidden weakness have considerably more resistance to a Trigger Event, but if you expose anyone to a powerful enough trigger event (e.g. the Bhopal explosion in India when a factory exploded exposing nearby residents to massive doses of dangerous chemicals), then they will become ill.

PART TWO

TREATING YOUR HAYFEVER

9

Conventional Medical Treatments for Hayfever

The present mainstream medical approach to hayfever often fails because it is based solely on using powerful drugs, such as antihistamines and steroids, that merely suppress the symptoms. The best way to cure allergies, including hayfever, is to try and identify the factors causing the hayfever, i.e. the neotoxins, and then to reduce the total load as much as possible. If symptoms still persist then it may be necessary to use medication. If you do take medication, it is important to get the maximum benefit with the minimum of side effects by taking it exactly as directed.

The symptoms caused by neotoxins such as pollen are often the body's attempt to heal itself. For example, the running eyes and nose of hayfever are the body's attempt to flush the offending pollen from the mucous membrane of the eyes and nose. Suppressing these compensatory mechanisms may easily direct the problem into another system. For example, when topical steroid creams are used to treat atopic eczema, the skin eruption often disappears but the problem is sometimes transferred to the lungs and increases the likelihood of asthma.

How Do Conventional Drugs Work?

To understand how drugs work, it is very helpful to have another look at the mechanism of classical hayfever (figure 9.1).

The key to treating hayfever successfully is to examine each of the stages in figure 9.1 to see how the hayfever process can be stopped at one or more points. The bulk of the information on how to carry this out is included in chapters 10, 11 and 12, but it is also very helpful to have a complete overview.

Figure 9.1: Mechanism of classical hayfever

Pollen	+	IgE antibody	+	Mast cell containing histamine	→	Pollen binds to antibody which attaches to mast cell membrane	→	Histamine release	→	Hayfever symptoms
naturally occurring protein		disturbed immune response								
A		B		C		D		E		F

Stage A: Pollen

It is worth stating the obvious. Classical hayfever cannot occur without pollen. This is the reason that sufferers are affected only during the months when pollen is released into the air. Although you may be a hayfever sufferer, if you can manage to avoid coming into contact with the pollen to which you are sensitive, then you will have no symptoms. You should plan to reduce your exposure to the specific pollens that affect you, both in place and time. In other words, where practical, don't walk near to plants to which you are allergic. Instead, stay indoors as much as is reasonably possible, keeping the windows closed and the pollen out. Secondly, when you take your summer holiday avoid contact with the plants that affect you by going to the seaside, or else to a foreign country where those plants are out of season. That way you'll remain symptomless.

Stages B + C: Immune System

It is a gross understatement to say that the immune system is complex and affected by a large number of factors. The IgE antibodies and mast cells are just a small part of the whole immune system which, along with the detoxification system, is affected by many types of neotoxins including infection, pollution of food, air and water, and stress. However, the most important part of the immune system in classical hayfever is the IgE antibody and the mast cell.

In most people, IgE is present only in tiny amounts, as opposed to the other classes of antibody (IgG, IgM and IgA), which are present at much higher levels. The main function of the IgE is to fight parasites. Not surprisingly, the blood level of IgE is often raised in people with parasitic infestations, particularly of the bowel.

The mast cell, described in chapter 1, is a special sort of white cell with a large nucleus and many granules of histamine. Due to a process called 'sensitization' which has occurred due to previous pollen exposure, a hayfever sufferer's body produces an excess of IgE specific to that pollen. When the same pollen reacts with the IgE antibody which is attached to receptor sites on the mast cell membrane, histamine granules are released into surrounding tissues. The disturbed immune response can often be normalized by attention to two complementary processes:

- reducing the 'total load' of pollution
- the right vitamin and mineral supplementation.

Stage B: Reducing the Effect of IgE Antibody

The IgE/mast cell reaction may also be reduced by a process known as 'desensitization'. This is carried out by injecting increasingly large amounts of the pollen to which the subject is allergic into the body. This induces production of a different type of antibody, called IgG, specific to that pollen. This desensitization process needs to be started well before the pollen season starts. In a patient who has been successfully desensitized, the usual hayfever reaction is blocked. Consequently, when pollen lands on the mucous membrane of the eyes and nose, instead of an IgE/mast cell reaction producing hayfever, the pollen is neutralized by the IgG and there are few or even no symptoms.

However, desensitization is not without risks. Occasionally a desensitization injection may set off a major allergic reaction, an anaphylactic shock (see page 23), which can be fatal. Consequently, desensitization is now rarely carried out except in specialized hospital allergy units with full resuscitation equipment immediately available.

Stages D+E: Stabilization of a Mast Cell Membrane
When the pollen attaches to the IgE antibody bound at the receptor site on the mast cell membrane, histamine is released.

If the mast cell membrane is 'stabilized' by a drug called sodium cromoglycate, then in spite of pollen and IgE antibody being present the histamine granules are not released.

Stage F: Blocking the Effect of Histamine
Histamine is a small protein which has its main effect on mucous membranes and tiny arteries. Its effects are described on p 22.

The histamine causes the early response. This consists of irritation and increased secretion of mucus and other fluids and occurs within 2-15 mins of exposure to the pollen. The late or delayed response causes swelling of eyes and nose and takes 4-12 hours to occur. Table 9.1 compares the early and late response.

Table 9.1: Comparison of early and late response on the nose

	EARLY RESPONSE	LATE RESPONSE
Time	2-15 min	4-12 hr
Caused by	Histamine	Neutrophils
Symptoms	Sneezing + running nose	Swelling
Treated with	Antihistamines	Steroids

DRUG TREATMENT OF HAYFEVER

The philosophy behind successful drug treatment of hayfever is to match the drug used with the severity of symptoms. There is a 'therapeutic ladder' of remedies available, starting with mild drugs which have a relatively minor effect on the body, working up to steroids taken by mouth or injection, which have a major effect on the metabolism of the whole body. As a good general rule, use the least powerful preparation that will remove the symptoms, although you may need to vary the dose according to the pollen count.

NB: It is very important to take the medication exactly as advised by your doctor/chemist and be aware of side effects such as sedation and special precautions and interactions, such as with alcohol, listed on the data sheet. If you have any concern about your illness or problems with treatment it is vital to contact a qualified practitioner *without delay*.

The therapeutic ladder starting with the least effective is listed below.

- Decongestants
- Antihistamines
- Membrane stabilizing drugs
- Local steroids
- Systemic steroids (systemic = relating to the body as a whole)

DRUGS USED IN THE TREATMENT OF HAYFEVER

All drugs are given three names:

- a chemical name, rarely used except by organic chemists
- an approved or generic drug name which is the same no matter who manufactures that particular drug
- a brand name, selected by the manufacturer for his product, which is usually by far the easiest of the three to remember.

The approved or generic name is the one used in the section below. If you are looking up the medication that you take for hayfever, you will find the approved name on the packaging, usually in small letters below the brand name. By reading the following sections, you will understand how it reduces your hayfever symptoms.

Decongestants
Drugs available as eye and nasal drops include: ephedrine, ipratropium bromide, oxymetazoline, phenylephrine hydrochloride, xylometazoline hydrochloride.

These drugs have a local effect and dry up the normal secretions of the nose and eyes. Apart from an initial improvement, in the long term they are usually unsuccessful for two reasons. Firstly, they deprive the nose of its normal protective layer of mucus. Secondly, when the decongestant is stopped, a rebound phenomenon occurs and there is an even greater level of secretion than occurred before treatment.

Antihistamines

1st generation antihistamines
  Highly sedative antihistamines: dimenhydrinate, promethazine, trimeprazine.
  Moderately sedating: chlorpheniramine, cyclizine, mequitazine.
2nd generation antihistamines
  Non-sedating: acrivastine, astemizole, cetirizine, loratadine and terferadine.

Antihistamines work by competing with histamines for the receptor sites on the linings of the mucous membrane and in the tiny blood vessels. This means that although histamine is released from the mast cell in the usual fashion, the antihistamine stops the hayfever symptoms from occurring.

The older first generation antihistamines often cause sedation, hence the warnings printed on these formulations such as 'This drug may cause drowsiness and should not be taken with alcohol. Care must be taken when driving, or operating machinery'. The second generation of drugs is usually as effective as the first generation preparations but rarely cause sedation.

Many Americans have a rather low opinion of over-the-counter antihistamine preparations because of the recommended dose previously written on the label was only half that usually be prescribed by a physician. Some antihistamines are long acting and taken only once a day. These should not be taken within the 24-48 hour period before going for skin testing. Although antihistamines are often quite successful in stopping the immediate histamine

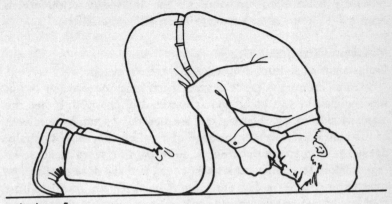

Bending down on floor

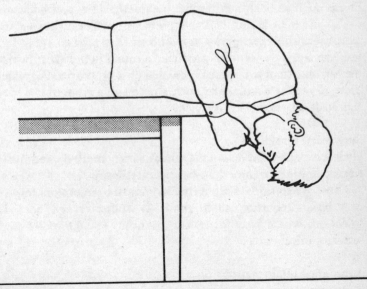

Using table or bed

Figure 9.2: Best position to use nasal spray

reaction, especially if taken before exposure to pollen, they have relatively little effect on stopping the delayed reaction which occurs 4–12 hours after exposure to an allergic challenge.

Membrane Stabilizing Drugs
Drugs such as sodium cromoglycate and ketotifen.

Sodium cromoglycate is a very inert substance which is not metabolized by the body, and is excreted unchanged. It has the effect of 'stabilizing' the mast cell membrane and stops the release of histamine even in the presence of a pollen that would usually cause the immediate reaction. Sodium cromoglycate needs to be taken before the pollen exposure occurs, and the dose needs to be repeated 4–6 times a day. Ketotifen is basically an antihistamine that has an effect resembling sodium cromoglycate.

Topical/Local Steroid Preparations
Drugs such as beclomethasone, betamethasone, and budesonide.

The mode of action of these preparations are discussed in the next section. Experiments have shown that a nasal spray formulated in aqueous solution produces a much better distribution of medication than the aerosol powered by a pressurized canister. In order to get the best results with a nose spray it should be used in the position shown in figure 9.2.

Systemic Steroids
Hydrocortisone, prednisolone, prednisone, methyl prednisolone, triamcinolone, dexamethasone, betamethasone.

These are steroids taken either by mouth or injection. Injections may be short-acting, up to about 24 hours, or else be a depot injection, which lasts for several months. The steroids have two separate effects:

- an anti-inflammatory
- an immunosuppressive effect.

The anti-inflammatory effect reduces the number of white cells migrating to damaged tissue, and also suppresses the effect of released histamines. The immunosuppressive effect decreases the level of circulating antibodies and reduces the white cell count.

Table 9.2: Table to show relative strength of different steroids

NAME	RELATIVE STRENGTH	DURATION OF ACTION
Hydrocortisone	1	Short Acting
Prednisolone	4	Short Acting
Prednisolone	4	Short Acting
Methyl Prednisolone	5	Short Acting
Triamcinolone	5	Moderate Acting
Dexamethasone	30	Long Acting
Betamethasone	30	Long Acting

Steroids should not be used in the long term because of serious side effects, which may affect long-term health, including:

- reducing resistance to infection
- thinning of the bone
- encouraging stomach ulcers, weight gain, diabetes and high blood pressure
- psychiatric symptoms
- withdrawal symptoms due to suppression of the usual steroid secretion by the adrenals.

Although steroids may be very useful in the short term, it is wise to avoid their long-term use, especially if they are taken systemically.

10

Food and Biological Neotoxins

An observer from outer space would be forgiven for thinking that the food industry's secret plan was to wage biological warfare on the population of the world. The increasing adulteration of food and drink with additives, hormones, antibiotics and many chemicals, together with the presence of food-borne infections, means that most people are digging a grave with their own teeth, and the vast rise in allergies and hayfever is completely understandable - even to be expected.

HOW DOES THE WRONG FOOD INCREASE THE RISK OF HAYFEVER AND ALLERGIES?

Polluted and non-organic food increases the risk of the eater suffering from hayfever and other allergies because it raises the *total load of neotoxins*. This increased load has a depressive effect on the immune and detoxification system which then reacts inappropriately to common and harmless proteins, like pollen, fungi, house dust mites, pet fur and food.

The function of this chapter is to expand on the brief introduction to biological neotoxins given in chapter 8 and give you some basic information that will help you beat your hayfever by diagnosing your food allergies.

SOURCES OF BIOLOGICAL NEOTOXINS

The sources of biological neotoxins include:

Food
This includes all edible matter and also all substances *deliberately* added to food, e.g. hormones, antibiotics, colouring, flavourings, preservatives and a host of others.

Although they will be mentioned in this chapter, all *food contaminants* (i.e. things that have found their way into food by accident, e.g. pesticides), will be dealt with in depth in the following chapter.

Water
Polluted water is a greatly under-recognized source of allergy. Despite reassurances to the contrary, an increasing number of people cannot drink tap water without becoming ill. Tap water is routinely treated with chlorine, sulphur dioxide, aluminium salts and fluorides, all of which may cause disease. Water contaminants (i.e. things that have found their way into the water by accident) will also be dealt with in the following chapter.

Infections
Infections are caused by bacteria, viruses, fungi or parasites, which may arise from the following sources:

infections present in food
infections present in water
infections caused by occupations

Animal Proteins

house dust mites
pets
other animals

Plant Proteins

tree pollen
grass pollen
weed pollen
fungi

FOOD

It is a scientific fact that the body completely replaces every molecule with a similar new one every 7 to 10 years. Consequently, if you eat heavily polluted food your body, especially your body fat, will become stuffed full of neotoxins due to an effect called bioaccumulation. This is the reason why the modern western diet increases the likelihood of suffering from hayfever and other allergic symptoms and diseases.

WHY DOES FOOD ALLERGY OCCUR?

There are several proposed explanations but one of the most widely accepted is:

Food allergy is caused by a failure of the body to adapt to the change in the human diet since the Stone Age.

To put it another way, we are giving our bodies the wrong food so they don't work properly. It is like putting diesel fuel in a petrol engine.

The human body was 'designed' to digest and live on the Stone Age diet. The essence of the Stone Age diet was *variety* and absence of neotoxins. Stone Age humans would eat everything that they could find that wasn't poisonous. This would include all sections of a plant from the roots at the bottom to the buds at the top, taking in stems, leaves, fruits, berries and nuts on the way. Equally, all non-poisonous animals were eaten, and not just a small variety of large mammals, chickens and a few species of fish as are eaten in the late 20th century. Instead, the Stone Age diet consisted of mammals both large and small, together with a wide variety of birds, reptiles and fish. Stone Age humans didn't eat just these animals listed above, which are all vertebrates, but would also eat a very wide variety of invertebrates including snails, shellfish, insects and worms.

Since the Stone Age, there have been three major changes in the diet:

- About 10,000 years ago humans ceased being nomads and settled down in one place cultivating wheat and other cereals. They also kept hens, and cattle, from which they got dairy products. Wheat products, eggs and dairy products were then eaten daily.
- Several hundred years ago sailing ships became faster; they were then used to import large quantities of common allergic foods like citrus fruits, tea, coffee, cocoa and sugar, which became available all the year round. Before this time, any fruit was available for only about three months of the year. In the absence of refrigeration, most foods couldn't be stored for more than a couple of months. Consequently, in the Stone Age, even if the food was gorged for three months, for the next nine months it was absent and couldn't be eaten until the next season came around.
- Since World War II the food industry has increased its output manifold by battery cultivation of animals and wide use of pesticides, fertilizers and petrochemical additives ('E numbers'). These petrochemical additives are now so widely added to improve food that it is difficult to have a diet completely free of colours, preservatives, antioxidants, emulsifiers or stabilizers.

As well as being chemically polluted, modern production methods yield food that, although looking attractive, contains abnormal amounts of vitamins, minerals, proteins, carbohydrates and fats. Food grown by these methods has been 'forced' to grow too rapidly and, consequently, it has much less vitality and health-giving properties than organic food. Worryingly, it has been reported that some oranges cultivated under intensive farming conditions in California contain no Vitamin C at all!

An increasing number of people become ill when they eat the modern diet which is repetitive and lacking in variety and giving high daily levels of the following: milk, cheese, butter, eggs, beef, wheat, wheat products, yeast, tea, coffee, cocoa, sugar, citrus fruits and additives. These particular foods are the most common cause of food allergy, especially the very high daily load of refined carbohydrates such as white flour and sugar which would have been almost completely absent from the Stone Age diet. The body cannot cope with an excessive volume or repetition of any one food and protests by exhibiting allergic symptoms and diseases, like hayfever.

WHICH FOODS ARE MOST LIKELY TO CAUSE AN ALLERGY?

Any food that is taken repeatedly may cause an allergy although some foods are highly allergic and are more likely to cause problems than others. Cooking tends to reduce the likelihood of allergy. This is because it 'fixes' large protein molecules breaking them down into smaller molecules, which are less likely to induce an immune response and are more easily processed by the detoxification system.

However, the substances most likely to cause allergy are highly fat soluble, (e.g. pesticides) which much prefer to remain in fat cell and brain rather than stay in the blood. These fat soluble chemicals can easily penetrate what is known as the blood/brain barrier to get into the brain. They also remain in the body for a very long time (10 to 40 years), since they are firmly bound to the fat stores. Since the average adult eats and drinks a ton of food each year, containing approximately 6 lb of food additives, even a small amount of pollution in a meal becomes a large amount when viewed cumulatively.

FOOD ADDITIVES

These are chemicals added to food to 'improve' the colour, flavour, shelf-life and marketability of the food products. Before World War II, relatively few food additives were used but in the western world it is now very difficult to get a diet that is completely free of additives. The best way to reduce your risk of hayfever and other allergies is to eat only fresh organic food and nothing from a packet or tin.

The mechanism by which food additives cause harm is at present poorly understood, but it appears that food additives disrupt the detoxification system by interfering with enzyme systems chiefly located in the liver, depleting the body stores of essential vitamins, minerals like magnesium and zinc, essential fatty acids and amino acids.

Some patients are highly susceptible to food additives, and as little as 1/10 teaspoonful of food containing an additive may be enough to set off a severe reaction. Tartrazine (E102) is one of the most dangerous additives and a very sensitive patient can sustain a severe allergic reaction after eating only a few micrograms (enough to cover the sharp end of a pin!)

A reaction may occur within seconds but often it will not show itself until after a delay of anything from 30 minutes to 24 hours. The outside limit for a reaction to show itself may be from 24 to 72 hours. As a general rule, the more severe the reaction, the more quickly it appears. Surprisingly, you may feel better after eating a food additive to which you are allergic because your allergy is said to be 'masked'. When you remove the same additive from your diet, it is usual to suffer withdrawal reaction that feels like a 'hangover' for the first 24 to 72 hours.

The food allergy lasts for as long as it takes the body to completely clear itself of the additive. It takes around 3 days for a food to completely pass through the bowel, and allergic symptoms may persist until the food is finally cleared.

You can usually tell if additives are present in a food by looking at the label. Manufactures are obliged by law to list all ingredients in their products in descending order of weight. However, there are several exceptions including 'take away' foods, individually wrapped sweets, unwrapped foods, alcoholic drinks with more than 1.2 per cent alcohol content, and medicines.

Unfortunately, reading the label is only useful up to a point. Sometimes, manufacturers are vague about an ingredient: for example, 'vegetable oil' could mean wheat oil, corn oil, soya oil, peanut oil or sunflower oil. An allergic patient might react to one of these oils but not to another, but without consulting the manufacturer has no way of knowing which one the food contains. Even this is not infallible, since manufacturers change formulations of their foods.

There is also the problem of 'hidden additives'. Many foods are made from ingredients that have already been processed themselves. For example, the main ingredient of cake is 'flour'. However, it is not possible to tell from the description 'flour' whether this ingredient contains any additives, e.g. bleaching agents, raising agents, colourings. A person allergic to 'flour' may not be reacting to the flour itself but to the unlabelled additives. Cake consists mostly of flour, and an additive put in during the flour processing can be present at a high level in the cake without warning.

DIAGNOSING FOOD ALLERGY

First, you must suspect that you have an allergy. See chapter 8 for details of the symptoms or diseases which may be caused by allergy. Allergy is greatly underdiagnosed. You can't find an allergy if you don't suspect it in the first place. Discovery depends upon the prepared mind.

The best way to find out which food(s) you are allergic to involves going on an exclusion diet (a diet containing very few foods and none of the common allergy-causing foods) to remove possible culprits, then 'challenging' yourself with the suspected foods, one at a time. You can do this yourself, although you will get by far the best results by consulting an Environmental Medicine practitioner. This method takes a bit of effort, but it is reliable and the results will be worth it.

NB: It is very important that before treating yourself you consult your doctor to make sure that you are not suffering from any undiagnosed condition that needs treatment. The testing works best if you are off all medication, including vitamins and minerals.

However, you must not stop prescribed tablets without the specific advice of your doctor. Bear in mind that medicines often contain additives, such as colourings and flavourings, and the bulk of the tablet is not an active ingredient but rather compacted milk sugar (lactose) or cornflour. If you are taking a prescribed medicine to which you are allergic, then the symptoms will not disappear on the exclusion diet.

PRE-TESTING

Fill in a diet diary (see below), for a week, writing down *everything* that you eat and drink including snacks.

Table 10.1: Diet Diary

Date:

Time	Food	Drink	Pulse Rate bpm	Symptoms 0–4	Comments
Breakfast					
Mid-morning					
Lunch					
Mid-afternoon					
Tea					
Supper					

Weigh yourself naked first thing in the morning (after emptying your bladder, and if possible after opening your bowels), and last thing at night.

Score your symptoms (hayfever or otherwise) *before* each meal, using the following scoring system:

0 = no symptoms   3 = severe symptoms
1 = mild symptoms   4 = very severe symptoms
2 = moderate symptoms

Also use the method of pulse testing. Take your pulse immediately before meals or snacks and count it for 60 seconds. Make sure you have been sitting still for at least two minutes before testing, and have not exerted yourself violently in the previous five minutes. Then following the meal take your pulse after 20 minutes, one hour and two hours, writing down the rate on the diet diary in the column marked 'Pulse Rate'. If your pulse rate goes up or down more than 20 beats a minute after a meal, then you should suspect that you have just eaten a food to which you are allergic.

It may seem surprising that the pulse rate can become faster or slower with an allergic reaction, but this is a common effect found in most organs. If a system (e.g. bowels) is undergoing an allergic reaction, it may be stimulated (diarrhoea) or suppressed (constipation), but in either case it does not work in the usual fashion. The reaction caused in the body is usually dose dependent. A small dose of neotoxin causes stimulation, but a larger dose causes suppression. The pulse test is a much more accurate indicator of allergy during the elimination diet and challenge stages.

When you have recorded your meals, pulse rate and symptoms, it may emerge that a particular food/drink makes you ill. You can avoid this food/drink when you start on the elimination diet.

EXCLUDING FOR ALLERGIC FOODS

This can be carried out in two ways.

a) The five-day fast. This involves eating no food at all for five days. The only thing taken is bottled spring water. However, most people in the western world are not used to fasting, and the five-day fast should not be carried out without the assistance of another responsible person. Ideally, it should be carried out under the supervision of a practitioner in Environmental Medicine, possibly in a specially equipped hospital ward.

b) The exclusion diet. This is a more practical proposition for people who are at work or with family commitments. An exclusion diet means coming off *all* the foods to which you are likely to be allergic for 7-10 days.

Most food allergic people react to more than one food. If you are allergic to four foods, your exclusion diet can be compared to a door with four bolts on it: you won't be able to open the door until *all* the bolts are drawn back. Similarly, you won't recover fully until *all* the allergic foods are removed from your diet.

On the day you start the exclusion diet it is a good idea to clear your bowel by taking the mild laxative Epsom Salts (magnesium sulphate). This will clear the bowel of food that you ate the day before you started the exclusion diet. You should take two teaspoonfuls of the Epsom Salts dissolved in half a pint of warm spring water. Smokers should make every effort to give up, or at least reduce their consumption to the minimum, since smoking is a massive cause of internal pollution and makes most allergies, including hayfever, worse.

Drink plenty of pure spring water from glass bottles as this will help to flush out the neotoxins. Spring water in plastic bottles should be avoided, since chemicals from the plastic are leached into the spring water, then absorbed.

Take plenty of exercise and arrange to take saunas three times a week whilst on the exclusion diet. The body excretes the neotoxin through sweat, whose production is greatly increased during exercise and saunas. There is no calorie restriction on the diet and there is no need for you to feel hungry. In spite of this, you are likely to lose about 7 pounds in weight during the exclusion period without feeling hungry. This weight loss occurs because a lot of retained water is lost as the allergy disappears.

Plan your meals in advance and buy only organic foods which are clear of chemicals and additives. Don't eat any processed food (i.e. anything in a packet or tin). If in doubt about a food or a food source, then leave it out. Be sure to read all the labels very carefully, since there are many 'hidden' foods. Highly allergic foods like milk, wheat or eggs are used in the preparation of a wide range of common foods. Unfortunately, these foods are often not clearly labelled and you may unwittingly find yourself eating something that is not permitted in your exclusion diet.

Self-catering is essential, since only then do you know precisely what you are eating. Don't eat in restaurants because you have no control over the ingredients used. Don't start an exclusion diet at a public holiday, i.e. Christmas, when dietary restriction will prove much more difficult. Use bottled water for drinking, washing food, cooking and brushing your teeth. When cooking, use steel or glass cooking utensils, don't use teflon non-stick pans, aluminium or plastic as chemicals leak out into the food. Don't eat food that has been wrapped in plastic or cling film. Don't use toothpaste; use bottled water on its own instead. Don't chew gum or take mints or non-prescribed medicines.

In order to beat your hayfever and allergies, it is essential to keep your diet diary as you did the preceding week. Continue to take your pulse before and after meals and weigh yourself in the morning and evening.

It is usual for you to feel worse for the first 3–4 days of the exclusion diet. This is the withdrawal reaction and feels like a hangover. You are particularly likely to crave foods to which you are allergic. However, don't give up, since taking even a small amount of a food to which you are allergic invalidates the exclusion diet and you will have to start again. Remember that 95 per cent compliance to the diet doesn't give 95 per cent improvement.

The common symptoms that you are likely to experience during the hangover period are:

- a severe headache, usually over the forehead
- a 'flu-like' illness without/with a slightly raised temperature
- marked irritability,
- feeling as though you are 'walking through treacle',
- feeling as though you are floating.

Fortunately, these symptoms rapidly pass, and then on days 5–9, provided that you have removed the appropriate foods, you should start to feel clear-headed with lots of energy and 'get up and go'.

Whilst you are on the exclusion diet, it is also important to reduce your *total load* of other neotoxins, i.e. chemicals, radiation and stress (see chapters 8, 11 and 12). Deciding which exclusion diet you should take is a difficult matter. Ideally it should be selected by an experienced practitioner of Environmental Medicine. The best exclusion diet for you will depend on your whole symptom picture.

There are two types of general exclusion diets which help a wide variety of allergic illnesses. The first is the Stone Age Diet (the Cave Man's Diet), which is the diet that humans have lived on for about nine tenths of their existence. The second is called the Oligoantigenic diet (Oligo = few), and this is made up of the few foods that are unlikely to cause food allergies.

The Stone Age Diet
This is an approximation to the largely carnivorous diet eaten by humans more than 10,000 years ago. It is cereal-free, dairy-free and chemical-free. One of the main reasons for the success of the Stone Age Diet is that it does not overload the body with large amounts of carbohydrates, which are the mainstay of the late 20th century diet. The human body seems to be far more able to deal with high protein and high fat intake, but not a high carbohydrate intake.

When eating the Stone Age diet, it is important for you to take a wide variety of the allowed foods. Don't just stick to meat and two vegetables. Providing that you eat a *wide* variety of the allowed foods then you can stay on the Stone Age diet indefinitely (as of course Stone Age people did).

Allowed

Fresh meats (organic if possible): beef, free range chicken, duck, goose, hare, partridge, pheasant, pigeon, pork, rabbit, turkey, venison.
Fish: all kinds, especially round fish (like cod) rather than flat fish (like plaice).
Fruit & vegetables: organic, without sprays or chemicals. Peel or wash in spring water before cooking in spring water.
Drinks: spring water in glass bottles
Seasoning: salt
Oils and margarines: sunflower and olive oil
Nuts: all kinds
Pulses: all kinds

Completely Avoid

Cereals: barley, bread and biscuits, corn, millet, oats, rice, wheat and all wheat products (these may be 'hidden')
Milk products: butter, cheese, cream, milk and yoghurt (these may be 'hidden')
Eggs (these may be 'hidden')
Sugars: chocolate and sweets, soft drinks, white and brown sugar
Processed foods: tinned meat & fish, crisps, processed nuts, bacon, smoked fish, kippers
Drinks: alcohol, coffee, tea
Chemicals: any packaged or processed food that contains chemicals

The Oligoantigenic Diet
These are selected from foods that are less likely to cause allergies. Dairy products, berries and nuts, pulses (legumes), and highly allergic cereals have been avoided. Take food from organic sources wherever possible.

Sample oligoantigenic diets

	DIET ONE	DIET TWO
Meat	Duck	Rabbit
Starch	Rice & rice flour	Potato & potato flour
Oils	Sunflower oil	Olive oil
Fruit	Grapes & grape juice	Peeled pears & pear juice
Vegetables	Carrots, parsnips & swedes	Broccoli, cauliflower, cabbage & sprouts
Other	Asparagus & apricots	Marrow & rhubarb

An Environmental Medicine practitioner will be able to give you ideas for other diets.

NB: The Oligoantigenic diets are for *short* term use, e.g. as an exclusion diet. Long term use is likely to cause deficiencies of vitamins, minerals and other food substances, and encourage allergies to develop to the few foods eaten.

CHALLENGE

Food allergy is confirmed if there is a big reduction in hayfever and other allergic symptoms when taking the exclusion diet. If you suffer from food allergy and you are taking the correct exclusion diet then an improvement in your health should have started by the 8th day, although an improvement in hayfever may take a lot longer. Ideally, the exclusion diet should be tried *before* the hayfever season starts. However, some conditions, like arthritis and eczema, take longer to improve. The arthritis and eczema exclusion diet should be prolonged for 10 or even 14 days.

Having confirmed a food allergy, it is necessary to identify which food(s) is responsible for the allergy. This is done by reinstating excluded foods into the diet. One new food is added every two days. The food challenging is done slowly because there may be a delay of up to 48 hours before a reaction becomes obvious.

There are some rapid reactions that occur after a short delay (¼ to 4 hours). These include pulse rate change, irritability and headache, lip swelling, vomiting and a runny nose. Urticaria, diarrhoea and asthma take longer to show (delay 1 to 24 hours) and the reaction that takes longest to show is usually eczema and arthritis (delay 6 to 48 hours).

When you a start a food challenge, you should initially take a small size portion one hour before lunch and then, if there is no reaction, a good size portion of the food at lunchtime. Eat only the food that you are testing. It is more difficult to tell a food reaction if you start the challenge food at breakfast, since many people feel less than their best in the morning. If you start the new food in the evening, the reaction may occur whilst you are asleep and be unnoticed. If you have no reaction at lunchtime, then take more of the same food at the evening meal and some more the next day. If you suffer no reaction during these two days then it is a 'safe' food and can be added to the foods already eaten.

When challenging yourself, it is wise to start with foods that are least likely to cause an allergic problem. Also, you should take foods as single ingredients: e.g. take wheat as a home-made biscuit containing only additive-free wholemeal flour, rather than bread which contains wheat, yeast and often additives. Fill in the results of your testing in the challenge sheet shown below.

Table 10.2: Results of Diet Diary

Date started	Food taken	REACTION (0–4)					
		DAY ONE			DAY TWO		
		AM	PM	EVE	AM	PM	EVE

If you have a reaction, then stop that food immediately. You may be able to reduce the severity of your allergic reaction by taking a tablespoonful of sodium bicarbonate (baking soda) in a pint of spring water. Most allergic reactions make the body more acid and this acidity can be neutralized by the sodium bicarbonate, which is a weak alkali. Your local chemist will be able to supply this substance to you without a prescription. Another helpful remedy is to take one gram of vitamin C (wheat free, milk free, and yeast free) with a large glass of water. The vitamin C helps the body's detoxification processes.

After a reaction you should not challenge yourself with another food until you get back to health. If you are unsure as to whether or not you reacted to a food, stop eating it for a week and then re-challenge yourself to the same food. In the interim try other foods. If you re-try the suspect food earlier than a week, the reaction may be 'masked' and consequently not show. Don't forget to challenge yourself with tap water as it is an increasingly common allergic substance.

You will probably find that different foods will give you different allergic symptoms with a different delay. For example, coffee may give you irritability and headache after a few hours, whereas wheat may give you arthritis after 24 hours. You should remember that most allergies are not fixed and can vary with time. One food that was previously harmless can give symptoms and encourage hayfever, especially after *trigger factors*, such as a virus infection, gastroenteritis, a shock, an operation, or a course of antibiotics.

Be sure to continue filling in your diet diary with your pulse rate and weigh yourself naked both in the morning and last thing at night. When you have an allergic reaction you may find that you fail to drop one to two pounds overnight because the allergic food causes water retention. Circle any allergy-producing foods in red.

OTHER WAYS OF DETECTING FOOD ALLERGY

There are several other methods of detecting food allergy which are used with varying degrees of success.

Skin Prick Testing

This is useful to detect inhaled substances that cause allergy, e.g. pollens, cat fur, house dust mite and fungi. Unfortunately, this method is not a reliable way to test for food allergies.

Blood Testing

In general, blood tests are not helpful in trying to identifying food allergies. The 'cytotoxic' test is of limited value and this is carried out by putting white cells from a patient's blood into weak solutions of foods. If the white cells shrivel, that probably indicates a food allergy.

Hair Testing

This is used for mineral content analysis of the body. Sometimes milk allergy is suggested by abnormal calcium and magnesium levels.

Applied Kinesiology

This is a test that uses principles of acupuncture. The theory of the test is that certain muscle groups become weak when the body is exposed to an allergic food. The weakness is judged by an observer who has to decide if the food has had an adverse effect. This method certainly deserves further study.

Provocation/Neutralization Test

This is carried out by injecting food extracts under the skin, or drops of the same into the mouth. Symptoms can be provoked and neutralized (removed) by giving food extracts of the correct dilution.

WILL MY FOOD ALLERGY BE PERMANENT?

Fortunately, the answer to this question is usually 'No'. Food allergy reaction can be divided into two types:

a) Fixed: this is due to an enzyme defect which is permanent. No matter how long food is avoided, it will always cause symptoms when it is taken (e.g. gluten contained in wheat causing coeliac disease).

b) Non-fixed or cyclical: this is much more common than the fixed kind. Recovery from a non-fixed food allergy can occur provided the food is avoided and that other allergy-producing foods and neotoxins (chemicals, radiation and stress) are kept to a minimum. A food allergy may not reveal itself if the total load of neotoxins is kept low. However, several neotoxins acting together can cause a far greater effect than the sum of their individual effects. The other important factor that encourages a non-fixed allergy to show itself is frequency of exposure to the food. If exposure to food is rare (less than once a week) then a food allergy is unlikely to arise.

Table 10.3: A typical 4-day rotary diet

Food	Day 1	Day 2	Day 3	Day 4
Protein	Fish	Lamb	Turkey	Rabbit
Fat/oil	Soya	Sunflower	Olive	Almond
Carbohydrate	Gram flour	Rice	Potato	Buckwheat
Fruit	Melon Pumpkin	Grapes	Banana	Apples/pears
Vegetables	Peas	Cabbage	Celery	Mango
	Beans	Cauliflower	Carrot	Spinach
	Lentils	Sprouts	Parsnip	Beetroot
Miscellaneous	Peanuts	Sultanas Raisins	Brazil nuts	Pistachio nuts
Drinks	Pineapple juice	Unfermented grape juice	Banana (liquidized)	Apple or pear juice

Table 10.4: Food Families

Food families are very useful ways of classifying foods. All members of a single food family are recognized by the body as being of similar origin. Someone who is allergic to one food is more likely to be allergic to other members of the same food family. Food families are of particular importance when designing exclusion and rotary diets. As a general rule, the further away from your home that a food grows, the less likely you are to be allergic to it. For example, rice grows in Asia, and rice allergy is rare in people who have lived in England all their life.

Food Families (Plants)

Banana family	banana
Beech family	chestnut
Borage family	borage, comfrey
Buckwheat family	buckwheat, rhubarb
Cactus family	prickly pear
Carrot family	carrot, celery, chervil, coriander, cumin, dill, fennel, parsley, parsnip
Cashew family	cashew nuts, mango, pistachio
Citrus family	grapefruit, kumquat, lemon, lime, orange, satsuma, tangerine
Composite family	artichoke, chamomile, chicory, dandelion, endive, globe lettuce, pyrethrum, safflower oil, sunflower (all forms), tarragon
Dillenia family	kiwi fruit (chinese gooseberry)
Fungi	alcohol, baker's yeast, mushrooms, vinegar, certain vitamins
Ginger family	cardomom, ginger, tumeric
Goosefoot family	beet, spinach, sugar beet
Gourd family	cantelope, courgettes, cucumber, gherkin, marrow, pumpkin, (water) melon
Grape family	grape, brandy, champagne, cream of tartar, raisin, sultanas, all wines, wine vinegar
Grass (western)	barley, corn (all forms), malt, maltose, oats, popcorn, sugar cane, wheat
Grass (eastern)	bamboo shoots, millet, sorghum, rice

Heath family	blueberry, cranberry, huckleberry
Honeysuckle family	elderberry
Laurel family	avocado, bayleaf, cinnamon
Legumes (also called pulses)	beans (blackeyed, butter, fava, green, haricot, lima, mung, navy, string), carob, chickpea, gum acacia and tragacanth, lentil, liquorice, pea, peanut, senna, soy bean, soya (all forms), tamarind
Lily family	Aloe vera, asparagus, chives, garlic, leek, onion, shallot
Maple family	maple syrup
Mint family	basil, lavender, lemon balm, marjoram, oregano, peppermint, rosemary, sage, spearmint, thyme
Morning Glory family	sweet potato
Mulberry family	breadfruit, fig, hop, mulberry
Mustard family	broccoli, Brussels sprouts, cabbage, cauliflower, chinese cabbage, horseradish, cale, mustard seed, radish, rape, swede, turnip, watercress
Myrtle family	cloves, eucalyptus, guava
Nutmeg family	nutmeg, mace
Olive family	olive and olive oil
Orchid family	vanilla
Palm family	coconut, date, sago
Papaya family	papaya
Passion Flower family	passion fruit
Pedalium family	sesame seed, tahini
Pepper family	peppercorn, black pepper, white pepper
Pineapple family	pineapple
Pomegranate family	pomegrante, grenadine
Potato family	pepper (Capsicum), cayenne, chili, paprika, potato, tobacco, tomato

Rose family	
1. *pomes*	apple, cider, cider vinegar, pectin, crab apple, pear, quince, rosehip
2. *stone fruits*	almond, apricot, cherry, nectarine, peach, plum, prune, sloe
3. *berries*	blackberry, loganberry, raspberry, strawberry
Sapodilla family	chewing gum
Sapucaya family	brazil nut, paradise nut
Saxifrage family	blackcurrant, currants, gooseberry, redcurrants, whitecurrants
Soapberry family	lychee
Spurge family	cassava, tapioca, castor bean
Sterculia family	chocolate, cocoa, cola nut
Tea	tea
Walnut family	English walnut, hickory nut, pecan
Yam family	Chinese Potato (Yam)

The following is a list of plants in which each case is the only member of a food family that is *commonly* eaten. Cross-sensitivity (reactivity with another member of the same family) is unlikely to occur with these foods:

avocado	ginseng	pineapple
banana	hazelnut	sweet potato
black pepper	juniper	sesame (tahini)
brazil nut	kiwi fruit	tapioca
chestnut	lychee	vanilla (natural)
elderberry	maple	yam
fig	olive	

Food Families (Animals)

MAMMALS

The Bovine Family

Beef	meat, rennet or rennin, sausage casings, suet
Milk	milk, butter, cheese, ice cream, lactose, yogurt, whey and caesin

| Goat | goats' milk, goats' cheese, goats' ice cream |
| Sheep | lamb and mutton, ewes' milk, ewes' cheese |

OTHER MAMMAL FOOD FAMILIES

Deer family	caribou, deer, elk, moose, reindeer
Hare family	hare and rabbit
Horse family	horse
Swine family	bacon, ham, lard, pork, sausage

BIRD FOOD FAMILIES

Duck family	duck and duck eggs, goose and goose eggs
Dove family	dove, pigeon
Grouse family	grouse and partridge
Pheasant family	chicken and chicken eggs, pea fowl, pheasant, quail
Turkey family	turkey and turkey eggs

FISH FOOD FAMILIES

Codfish	cod, coley, haddock, hake
Flatfish	dab, flounder, halibut, plaice, sole
Herring	herring, pilchard, sardine
Mackerel	mackerel, skipjack, tuna
Salmon	salmon, trout
Molluscs	clam, mussel, oyster, scallop, snail, squib
Crustacean (Shellfish)	crab, crayfish, lobster, prawn, shrimp

The following animals are the only members of their food family that are *commonly* eaten. Allergy is unlikely to occur due to cross-activity without another member of the same food family:

| anchovy | rabbit | turkey |
| deer | sturgeon | whitefish |

Long-Term Dietary Modification

An exclusion diet (see above) is a good way to identify your food allergy, but it will cause deficiency diseases if it is the sole form of nutrition long term. In addition, a repetitive restricted diet, in the long term, is likely to cause food allergies to the new foods taken.

The answer to this problem is the *rotary diet* which is a way to prevent emergence of new allergies and maintain tolerance to those foods excluded. The easiest way to understand a rotary diet is to see a typical one (table 10.3).

Table 10.3 shows a four-day Rotary Diet. After day 4, the diet rotates back to day one, hence the name. The principle is that no food is eaten more frequently than every four days, and no 'food family' is repeated more often than every two days. In order for you to plan your own Rotary Diets successfully, it is essential to consult the table of food families given in table 10.4.

There are a few other important points. Always eat organic foods that have not been processed, sprayed with chemicals, tinned or packaged. Be obsessive about reading labels and finding out the ingredients of everything you eat. Remember that some foods may be 'hidden'. Run your diet day from 4.00 pm to 4.00 pm and that way your lunch and evening meal will be in different diet days, and consequently you will have more variety of food in a day.

BOWEL FLORA AND ITS EFFECT ON ALLERGIES

The bowel is normally filled with billions of yeasts and bacteria that in health exist in a self-regulated balance. Their function is to produce vitamins and act as a initial first stage in the detoxification process before the liver. Their chemical flexibility is remarkable and they are able to break down almost any molecule thrown at them.

Consequently, there are major consequences when the bowel flora are altered. The common factors causing an alteration in bowel flora include drugs and diet.

- Antibiotics – especially broad spectrum antibiotics given for a protracted period.
- Steroids – hydrocortisone, prednisone, prednisolone and also the sex steroids in the oral contraceptive pill.
- Sugar – excess sugar and carbohydrates encourage growth of yeast.
- Alcohol and yeast-containing foods – encourage growth of yeasts.

Any factor that changes the gut flora is likely to produce the following.

- Intralumenal change: The lumen is the cavity of the gut along which the food passes. Loss of the normal detoxification capability and vitamin production causes production of gas, diarrhoea and poisons such as acetaldehyde.
- Bowel wall changes: The build up of poisons in the lumen of the bowel damages the cells of the gut which no longer dissolve certain important nutrients, and fail to keep out undigested foods and other poisons normally excluded.
- Body changes: The immune system and liver detoxification system become overwhelmed with undigested food molecules which are recognized as 'foreign' and attack. Poisons like acetaldehyde are dissolved in levels greater than can be detoxified and other 'rogue' molecules have hormone-like effects and many even affect DNA and other enzyme proteins.

WATER

There are several ways in which water can induce environmental illness.

Infections

Waterborne infections are becoming more, rather than less common. These occur in drinking water, rivers and on beaches.

'Normal' water processing
During domestic water processing chemicals are added which
include aluminium salts, chlorine, fluoride and sulphur dioxide.
The section in this chapter will look at the effects of chemicals that
are deliberately added to water.

Water Contaminants
These are chemicals that have found their way into the water by
accident. The sources of these chemicals include industrial
manufacturing processes, agricultural chemicals and the lining
of water pipes. These will be dealt with comprehensively in
chapter 11.

INFECTION

Infections are important in Environmental Medicine because
although they are not allergies themselves, they can frequently
trigger allergies. Bowel infections in infants are the commonest
cause of allergies starting in children aged 0 to 2 years.

Infections trigger allergies by damaging enzyme systems and
making cell membranes more permeable, overloading the immune
and detoxification systems, which in an allergic patient are already
busy trying to deal with neotoxins (see figure 10.1).

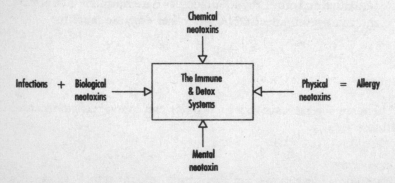

Figure 10.1

Allergic symptoms commence when the total load of neotoxins exceeds the threshold of the immune and detoxification systems' ability to cope. The total load, however, varies unpredictably from day to day, which explains the variability of allergic symptoms.

There are two ways of avoiding infection:

General
Reduce your total load of neotoxins. This reduces the burden on your immune and detoxification systems and improves your general health, making you much more able to fight infections successfully.

Specific
Alter your lifestyle so that you reduce your exposure to infections as much as possible. The following section will give you details about some of the more important infections from food and water.

As with most infections, it is the very young, the old and those whose immune system is not working properly who will first become ill. However, a healthy person often shows no symptoms of minor infections although the immune system will be put under strain.

Chemical Neotoxins

Hayfever is a paradox! Despite the fact that the pollen count is dropping, the incidence of hayfever is still rising. In a nutshell, the reason for this is the increasing level of pollution of air, food and water, which causes an increase of both classical IgE/Mast cell hayfever and non-specific rhinitis, which is really a variety of 'chemical sensitivity' which may mimic hayfever.

This chapter will introduce you to the concept of chemical sensitivity and help you diagnose and treat it. By reducing your problem with chemicals, you will probably be able to reduce your frequency and severity of hayfever symptoms.

The reason that we are suffering such massive problems with chemical sensitivity is that there are so many sources of chemical pollution. There are now over 350 million cars in the world, and factories all round the globe are releasing fumes and making products that release chemicals into the atmosphere, e.g. paints, glues, plastics, aerosols and solvents. We are reaching (or have passed) the planet's capacity to recycle all these chemicals.

But what is worse is that chemical fumes don't just stay where they are created or sprayed. The alarming results of tests have shown that when a pesticide is sprayed in North Africa on a Monday, some of it reaches London by Wednesday and another portion reaches Florida by Friday. The good news is that we have a large number of environmental groups who are making big efforts to save the rainforests, endangered species and the whale. Fortunately, what is good for the planet is also good for the individual and helps to reduce the incidence of allergic disorders including hayfever.

The way that you are helping yourself and others is to reduce your own total load of neotoxins, which will assist to reverse the downward spiral. Chemical pollution is particularly an area where we must *think globally but act locally.*

Apart from the effect chemicals have on your total load of neotoxins, very possibly making them a factor in your hayfever, many people are more obviously sensitive to chemicals. These problems are more accurately called sensitivities rather than allergies, though the latter term is still frequently used. Chemical sensitivities usually start because of one source of chemicals, e.g. car fumes. If this neotoxin is not removed then the body starts to react to other chemicals as well (see page 71). These are called 'cross sensitivities'. If exposure continues, the number of cross sensitivities increases still further until the body reacts to almost every food and chemical in the environment. This is the stage where a person is called a 'universal reactor'.

Chemical sensitivity can be triggered by two sorts of chemical events.

1. Acute Massive Exposure

This may occur after an industrial accident (**reported** events include Bhopal in India, Soweso in Italy and Flixborough in England), chemical application and handling (e.g. pesticides spraying or chemical spill), or wartime exposure (mustard gas, nerve gas, Agent Orange). If you experience an acute massive exposure to chemicals you will almost certainly remember it because of the drama surrounding the event, but sensitivity may persist permanently after the exposure.

2. Chronic Exposure

Chemical sensitivities usually start due to chronic exposure to a chemical neotoxin, e.g. formaldehyde. The standard, but **incorrect** advice, is that there can be no danger because the concentration of the chemical is below the officially recognized danger level, which has been set at a far too high a level. As time progresses the vast majority of these safe levels are revised downwards.

The 'safe' level of a chemical is often completely wrong because of four fundamental errors in the testing processes.

(i) Wrong Individuals Tested

Chemical toxicity testing is carried out on healthy volunteers (usually young men), when those most susceptible are the very young or old, pregnant women and those already ill. Other toxicity tests carried out on laboratory animals, e.g. rats, yield questionable results because of major differences between human and other mammals' metabolism, e.g. rats can make their own vitamin C.

(ii) Acute Testing but Chronic Exposure

The toxicity testing is usually carried out over a relatively short period, despite many individuals' chronic exposure. A chronic exposure allows chemicals to bioaccumulate and after many years they may reach dangerous levels and cause symptoms.

(iii) Individual Variation Ignored

There is enormous individual variation from person to person in the ability to detoxify any chosen chemical. A standard dose of chemical that has no obvious effect on one person will make another very ill (as in the different effect of alcoholic drinks on different people). Individuals who have defective detoxification systems are much more likely to suffer from chemical sensitivity.

(iv) 'The Cocktail Effect'

In the real world we are exposed to hundreds of different chemicals every day. A chemical on its own may be relatively harmless, but when mixed with other commonly occurring chemicals may cause an interaction that makes it much more toxic, e.g. alcohol and tranquillizers.

Another problem is that many organic chemicals are bound to body fat, and over time the amount stored goes up due to an effect called bioaccumulation. The body is often not able to excrete the chemical in the times between exposures and thus the level continually goes up over your whole lifetime. Chronic exposure is particularly likely to be a problem if your total load of neotoxins is also high.

WHAT HAPPENS WHEN I AM EXPOSED TO A CHEMICAL NEOTOXIN?

On the initial exposure to a chemical neotoxin you will usually suffer an 'alarm reaction'. Common symptoms include light-headedness, headache and palpitations, and you will be able to smell the chemical.

If exposure continues the 'adaption phase' is entered: your body gets used to the neotoxin and sense of smell for that chemical is lost. Surprisingly, instead of feeling unwell, continuing exposure to the chemical may often give you a 'lift' (e.g. glue sniffing). If exposure then ceases, as the level of the chemical in the body drops, then withdrawal symptoms begin, mimicking a hangover.

If, instead of removing the chemical, exposure continues, eventually you will reach the 'exhaustion stage', and instead of a chemical giving you a 'lift', you will feel immediately worse at each new exposure. By this time there may well be permanent damage to the body.

HOW CAN I TELL IF I HAVE A CHEMICAL SENSITIVITY?

There are particular features that will suggest you have a chemical sensitivity.

- You may have many symptoms, especially headache, fatigue, reduced concentration and memory, muscle weakness, irritability, excitability and feeling 'doped up'. Any or all of these symptoms are likely to come on after the initial exposure, or else during the 'hangover'.
- You are likely to be chemically sensitive to several different

groups of substances, e.g. combustion fumes, solvent fumes, plastic fumes, formaldehyde, alcohol and antibiotics.

- You will probably feel worse in one particular place, e.g.in the kitchen, or at one particular time, e.g. on Mondays when returning to work, or on long car journeys. Often other people will feel unwell in the same place.
- You feel better outdoors and in well ventilated places.
- You dislike, or paradoxically are very fond of chemical fumes, e.g. petrol fumes, tar fumes, glue and paint fumes.
- You are likely either to have a very acute sense of smell or to have lost your sense of smell completely.

WHAT FACTORS MAKE A CHEMICAL SENSITIVITY MORE LIKELY?

A High Total Load of Neotoxins
If your load of neotoxins from **all** sources, i.e. biological neotoxins, (food, water, infection), chemical neotoxins, physical neotoxins (electromagnetic radiation, sound) and mental neotoxins, (stress, life changes and accidents) is high then you're more likely to suffer a chemical sensitivity. It is the **total** load that is important, since that governs how much reserve your immune and detoxification systems have left.

Your Individual Susceptibility
This is dependent on your age, your sex, your racial background and the genes that you were given by your parents. As a general rule, young children and old people have less resistance to most problems. Adult women seem to be about twice as likely as men to suffer from allergies, although before puberty allergies seem to be commoner amongst boys.

There is a large genetic variation in the ability to withstand exposure to chemicals. This is related to the activity of liver and other enzymes systems. Some people produce defective enzymes and consequently, the body is not able to process certain neotoxins, making such individuals much more susceptible to chemical sensitivities. There is no obvious outward sign that susceptible people have a problem. However, the speed at which an individual can break down standard doses of the drug debrisoquine, and the amino acid carboxymethy-cysteine, gives a good idea of the individual's resistance to chemical sensitivity.

Your Resources for Recovery
Recovery from most chemical insults can be achieved with further avoidance of chemicals, the right diet, sleep and rest, exercise (and also saunas to encourage loss of toxins through sweat), and appropriate vitamins and mineral supplements.

HOW DO CHEMICALS ENTER THE BODY?

Chemicals enter the body through three routes: by being eaten, by being inhaled or by contact with the skin.

Chemical Neotoxins in Food and Drink
There are many contaminants in food and water. They have got in by accident or by bad practice. These chemicals are absorbed through the bowel, which has a surface area of 400 square metres, and may affect any organ.

Common chemical contaminants in food include halocarbon and hydrocarbon solvents; insecticides, herbicides and fungicides; antibiotics, hormones and steroids; petrochemical fuels oils and waxes and their breakdown products; metals and plastics from cooking utensils; phenolic compounds including tin can linings; formaldehyde compounds; natural gas and other gases.

Chemical contaminants in tap water include halocarbons and hydrocarbon solvents; other halocarbons, including PCB; insecticides, herbicides and fungicides; nitrates and other fertilizers; heavy metals including lead, mercury, cadmium, aluminium, copper and arsenic; polyvinyl chloride; sex steroids; asbestos; infections from sewage disposal and contamination by animal manures and household waste; and toxic gases such as sulphur dioxide.

There is an effect called *bioconcentration* that occurs with chemicals that are stored in body fat, e.g. pesticides. The result of this effect is that these substances become more concentrated as they pass up the food chain. Since people are always at the end of food chains (no animal eats humans), we are the ones who experience the worst effects of this phenomenon. The concentrating effect along a food chain can be as much as 100,000 times! Mother's breast milk, which is largely an emulsion of fat, further concentrates poisons stored in fats, which is why it is vitally important that a nursing mother should have an unpolluted diet.

The way to avoid chemical contamination of food is to eat organic food; failing that, natural food, fresh and without additives, but certainly avoid junk food. The way to avoid chemical contamination of water is to drink a spring water recommended by your Environmental Medicine practitioner from a safe source in glass bottles (water in plastic bottles contains chemicals leached from the plastic). Even spring water is only as pure as the source and the bottling method. There are many ways of purifying water. The method chosen depends on which contaminants that you are trying to remove. No single process is best for all problems.

Always run your water for 2 to 3 minutes if water has stood overnight in pipes. Lead levels can be 100 times higher than normal after overnight standing, especially in soft water areas.

Inhalation
The fastest and commonest way for chemicals to enter the body is through the lungs. The lungs have a very large surface area equivalent to that of half a tennis court (100 square metres). This enables chemicals to enter the blood's circulation within 1 to 2 seconds and to get to the brain in 7 seconds, hence the very rapid effect of airborne chemicals especially on the brain.

Skin Contact
The skin provides a large surface area for the absorption of

chemicals (1.5 square metres). More than half of the chemicals entering the body from water are absorbed through the skin. However, the chemicals that are most easily absorbed through the skin are those that are fat soluble, i.e. most organic chemicals.

WHICH CHEMICALS ARE LIKELY TO CAUSE PROBLEMS WITH MY HEALTH AND HAYFEVER?

There are so many chemicals that it is necessary to have some sort of classification of these substances. A loose classification based on the use of the chemical is far more valuable than a precise but unmanageable scientific classification based on chemical composition. Consequently, there is considerable overlap in the following list.

- petrol and diesel and their combustion products
- natural gas, other fuels and their combustion products
- incinerators
- cigarette smoke
- solvents and glues, paints and varnishes ('do it yourself')
- cleaning fluids and polishes
- pesticides (insecticides, herbicides, fungicides)
- fertilizers (nitrates)
- pharmaceutical drugs
- dyes
- plastics
- synthetic fibres and materials
- soaps and detergents
- perfumes, cosmetics and deodorants
- treated papers, boards and woods (chipboard & plywood)
- chlorinated hydrocarbons (halocarbons with C-Cl bond)
- toxic gases (sulphur dioxide, oxides of nitrogen, ozone)
- toxic metals (lead, mercury, cadmium, arsenic, aluminium)
- alcohols (all alcoholic drinks, surgical & methylated spirits)
- phenols (dyes, drugs, plastics, preservatives)

- terpenes (paint fumes, anaesthetics, hydrocarbon fuel fumes)
- formaldehyde (textiles, dyes, foams & rubbers, & many others)

Petrol, Diesel and Their Combustion Products (Motor Vehicle Fumes)
We are now starting to pay the price for the motor car age. The centres of most large cities are no longer fit for human habitation due to the alarmingly high level of petrol and diesel fumes. Petrol and diesel fumes are amongst the commonest causes of chemical sensitivity. They are the main cause for the increase in hayfever over the past 30 years. Pointers that suggest that your chemical sensitivity problem may be due to car fumes include:

- being ill in cars and buses, especially when sitting in the back with the window open.
- being unwell when you go into the centre of a town, especially in the rush hour.
- living near a busy road, especially one with a junction or underpass where car fumes build up. People living near a busy road have been found to have a raised incidence of cancer.

If you have a chemical sensitivity to vehicle fumes you should move away from a main road to a less busy one. To assess whether or not you are too close to a main road, you should use the general rule that if you can **hear** traffic, then you are too close.

One of the commonest ways to induce chemical sensitivity and increase hayfever risk is to have a house with an integral garage. The chemical sensitivity arises when exhaust fumes leak into the house. It may also be due to other DIY chemicals kept in the garage. The garage is often used to store paints, solvents, varnishes, glues and cleaners which, even if sealed, still tend to leak a little. Petrol exhaust fumes are hot and, therefore, rise, consequently, the room above the garage (often a bedroom) becomes filled with these gases. If the occupant of that room also has a poor diet and stressful lifestyle (high total load of neotoxins), then a chemical sensitivity is very likely to arise.

The ingredients of traffic fumes are not just hydrocarbons but also oxides of nitrogen and carbon monoxide. When these gases are exposed to bright sunlight, ozone and free radicals are formed, which once again add to the total load that must be managed by the detoxification system.

Natural Gas, Paraffin, Heating Oil and Their Combustion Products (Central Heating and Cooking)

These are used to heat homes, offices and schools. Chemical sensitivity may arise from the unburnt fuels or their combustion products. Some patients are so sensitive to natural gas that there is enough leakage from existing plumbing, even when all devices are turned off, to give them symptoms. The effect of the leakage is made worse because natural gas rises (through being lighter than air) and also it is supplied at higher pressure than the previously used town gas.

An unventilated kitchen is a potentially dangerous place to be. Natural gas combustion fumes contain carbon monoxide and oxides of nitrogen. After a gas cooker has been burning for a couple of hours in an unventilated kitchen, the level of pollution with toxic gases is several times higher than that experienced standing in busy rush hour traffic. This is a very good reason to ensure that when you're in your kitchen you open a window and/or turn on your extractor fan.

Some chemically sensitive people react to food cooked in a gas oven. It sometimes occurs that people with an apparent coffee allergy are not, in fact, allergic to the coffee but to the gas used to roast the coffee beans.

Unburnt paraffin liquid and especially paraffin combustion fumes cause problems in susceptible people. Paraffin fires are usually put in the centre of a room without any proper escape route for the exhaust gases, and toxic fumes are likely to build up to dangerous levels.

Central heating system design and installation often leaves a lot to be desired. The flues are sometimes placed in areas where fumes can leak back into the house. Chemical sensitivity to central heating fumes is usually worse in the winter, and inside the house, and better in the summer and outside the house. The best heating for allergic people is movable electric radiators providing, of course, that they are not electrically sensitive. With a chemically sensitive person, if a gas central heating boiler is used it should be sited in a sealed room that does not directly communicate with the house. This prevents leakage of burnt and unburnt fumes into the house affecting the occupants.

Incinerators

Incinerators are used to dispose of dangerous chemicals like PCBs and contaminated organic solvents by burning them at high temperatures. Even when they are working properly, residents in surrounding areas are showered with neotoxins and carcinogens. If the incinerator is operated at a lower temperature, then horrendously poisonous chemicals like dioxins are produced and this explains the high incidence of allergies and cancer in the proximity of such incinerators. Even incinerators processing ordinary domestic waste give off toxic fumes.

Cigarette Smoking

Smoking is a major preventable cause of ill health and the most important cause of premature death (dying before the age of 65 years) in the western world. Exclusion diets, avoidance of chemicals and other measures you may undertake in order to lessen your symptoms of hayfever or other allergies are of reduced value in smokers or passive smokers (non-smokers breathing in other people's smoke). Cigarettes contain nicotine and tar, both of which have a damaging effect on the immune system.

Solvents, Glues, Paints and Varnishes (Do It Yourself)

It has long been known that the vapour of solvents and glues, paints and varnishes may bring on an asthma attack. However, any of the above chemicals may be responsible for symptoms of chemical sensitivity, and they also increase your total load of neotoxins. Unless you work with the above chemicals, exposure is usually episodic and easier to relate to a bout of illness. However, highly susceptible individuals will react to very low levels of 'DIY' products e.g. leakage from storerooms and garages. Even the apparently tightly sealed bottles and cans often leak a little.

When you are painting or gluing in an enclosed space, you will usually receive a massive dose of halocarbon (chlorine-carbon bond) solvents. All the solvent must fully evaporate from a glue, paint or varnish for it to harden into its long-lasting form. Since there is no escape route for the solvent in an enclosed space with poor ventilation, the atmospheric concentration builds up rapidly. The high concentration means that solvent is then inhaled and absorbed into the body through the lungs.

Cleaning Fluids and Polishes
Under this heading is included a wide range of cleaning fluids, carpet and 'dry' cleaners, and a range of wood, floor and metal polishes. These all contain halocarbon solvents which are fat soluble and are absorbed very quickly through the lungs and skin. They have their greatest effect on the brain which is made largely of fat. Consequently most of the symptoms caused by these substances are mental (e.g. irritability, and muscle weakness).

Pesticides
Pesticides are a particularly important type of chemical sensitivity since they give symptoms that are somewhat labelled as 'hayfever' or flu. In fact, a lot of these sort of symptoms develop due to the highly toxic nature of the chemicals involved.

These substances have been designed to be poisonous in very low concentrations and 1 teaspoonful can kill an adult. Plants and animals have great difficulty in breaking down these substances and, consequently, pesticides persist in the environment for many years. However, the pesticides don't stay where they are sprayed. They travel thousands of miles in air currents, and are leached in to the water supply, at which point they enter the food chain.

They are bioconcentrated along food chains (see page 126), and there is often a long delay between application to the ground and the side effects of poisoning becoming obvious in the plant and animals in the food chain. Even if use of pesticides stopped today, it would be another 30 years before we would see the full effect of the pesticides that have already been applied.

There is also the phenomenon of 'synergy' (a magnification effect) between pesticides. This means that when two pesticides are used together, their combined effect may be 100 times greater than using one or other on its own. Synergy may also occur between a pesticide and its 'inert' base. The deadly dioxin may be present in a pesticide without notification, increasing the poisonous effect on flora, fauna and humans. The usage of pesticides has increased 5 to 15 times since usage began because the pests sprayed have become resistant. However, another problem is that the predators that fed on the pests have also been killed. Despite regulations governing use, there is little *practical* control over how, when and where pesticides are applied. Governments don't routinely measure pesticide levels. This is probably because they would have to take some action when they were found to be too high.

Pesticides 'bioaccumulate' in body fat. It may take several years of chronic exposure to a pesticide before symptoms start to appear. The symptoms usually will not start to lessen until detoxification is carried out. The threshold for symptoms can vary daily depending upon general health level.

Pesticides can be classified according to their usage:

---

a) **Insecticides**
These are used to kill insects that feed on crops. They are used on *growing* crops and consequently are likely to be incorporated into the plant tissue. They are also used to treat stored grain. There are four groups of insecticides:
(i) **organochlorine** - very persistent fat bound pesticide.
(ii) **organophosphorus** - derived from nerve gases.
(iii) **carbamates** - work in a similar way to organophosphorus compounds.
(iv) **pyrethroids** - initially derived from the chrysanthemum plant.

b) Herbicides

There are two sorts of herbicides:

(i) non-specific ones that kill all plant life.

(ii) specific ones that kill broad leaved plants, i.e. weeds, leaving the crop unharmed.

Some herbicides have a similar structure to naturally occurring plant hormones and growth promoters. These are absorbed into the plant and then either block metabolism or wildly overstimulate it, in either case causing plant death.

c) Fungicides

These kill fungi and they are usually based on a heavy metal, e.g. mercury or copper, or a hydrocarbon compound containing sulphur. They are sprayed on plants, especially fruit, and they are often applied with paraffin to promote penetration into the tissue. At the time of eating traces of fungicides can still be found in food and, unfortunately, washing does not remove these chemicals.

Fungicides are also used to preserve wood and kill dry rot. Pentachlorophenol (PCP) is a major health hazard to the workers making and using it. Despite the insistence of building societies and banks on fungicidal treatment of houses, it is often not necessary. Wood used in construction of houses remains strong for up to 500 years providing that it is kept dry and well ventilated. There are now low toxicity fungicides that have a 10 year life as opposed to the usual 30 year life, and are much less poisonous.

Fertilizers (Nitrates)

Plants require nutrients from the soil before they can grow. One of the essential nutrients is nitrogen. Only a small proportion of the nitrogen in the soil is free (inorganic nitrogen NO_3) and available for plant growth. The rest is bound in decaying plants and animal manure. Plant growth can be accelerated dramatically by putting nitrate (NO_3) or ammonia (NH_3) fertilizer on the soil. However, only about half of the applied nitrate fertilizer is taken up by the growing plant. The other half is leached out by rain and surface water. After a long delay, of up to 20 or 30 years, the fertilizer finds its way into drinking water. The present nitrate level in drinking water reflects the application of fertilizers a generation ago. The nitrate level in drinking water is likely to rise 2 to 3 times in the early part of the 21st century.

The nitrate in water is converted to nitrite by bacteria in the mouth. This causes several problems: nitrites combine with haemoglobin (the red pigment in blood), to form the blue pigment methaemoglobin. Babies are particularly vulnerable to this change and nitrites can cause the 'Blue Baby Syndrome', which may be life threatening. Nitrites also encourage the development of stomach cancer.

Pharmaceutical Drugs
Pharmaceutical drugs that have powerful effects also have the capacity to produce powerful side effects. There is even a condition with hayfever-like symptoms called drug-induced rhinitis (see chapter 7). Half of the British population are particularly vulnerable to drug-induced side effects because they have slightly defective liver enzymes and are what is called 'slow acetylators' (i.e their liver enzymes can only break down certain drugs slowly). This half of the population are more likely to suffer from drug-induced side effects, e.g. rashes, nausea and drug-induced rhinitis.

The very young and the old are more likely to suffer from drug-induced side effects. This is because their livers and other enzyme systems are less efficient than those of the young and middle aged.

Iatrogenic diseases (diseases caused by doctors giving too high a dose or giving the wrong drug) are, unfortunately, very common (probably at least 1 in 10 of all illnesses). One of the first measures often tried when admitting a confused pensioner to hospital is to take him or her off all medication. A large proportion get dramatically better.

Drugs are made up of two parts: the active ingredient, and the base (the filler used to make up the weight), which contains additives. Sometimes, the problem caused by a drug is not related to the active ingredient but to the base or the additives (colourings, flavourings and preservatives). Some allergic patients react to the lactose (milk sugar), or cornflour used as a base. Others react to the additives. Until recently, a well-known antihistamine tablet which was used to treat allergic conditions contained tartrazine (E102), which is a frequent cause of allergic reactions.

Dyes

Dyes are a major cause of allergies and sensitivities. By far the biggest source of the problems are azo dye food additives which have no nutritional value but are used to 'improve' the appearance of food. Azo food dyes particularly affect individuals who are already allergic to aspirin. About one fifth of aspirin sensitive people are also allergic to azo dyes and these individuals are usually middle aged or older, and more commonly women than men.

Fabric dyes may also cause chemical sensitivities, especially aniline and chromate dyes. As a general rule, the lighter the dye and the more natural the source, the less likely it is to cause problems.

Plastics

These synthetic substances affect chemically sensitive people due to 'outgassing', (i.e. release of gases including formaldehyde and plasticizers). As a general rule, the harder the plastic, the less outgassing that occurs. The older plastics like Bakelite and Formica are usually safe. However, the modern *soft* plastics are much more likely to cause a problem. As a general rule, if you can mark them with your fingernail or smell them they are more likely to give you a problem.

The worst plastics for outgassing are polythenes (plastic containers) and polyvinyls (plastic curtains, upholstery and pipes), silicone seals, epoxy glues, polyurethane foams and stuffings, and teflon kitchen utensils.

Synthetic Fibres and Fabrics

You may be allergic to synthetic fibres and fabrics because these both release formaldehyde. If your chemical sensitivity is caused by synthetic fibres and fabrics, then you can remain in good health by dressing in natural fabrics, e.g. cotton and wool. (Check that the wool or cotton have not been treated with pesticides.) Large areas of synthetic fibres may also be found in curtains, carpets, upholstery, wall coverings and bed clothes. The worst fibres for outgassing formaldehyde are polyesters.

Soaps and Detergents

Natural soap made without perfume is generally safe. However, the modern detergents are manufactured from petrochemicals and may give problems. Especially bad are 'biological' powders containing enzymes. After a machine wash there is quite enough detergent left in clothes to produce symptoms in susceptible individuals.

Skin irritation is the commonest problem occurring with detergents. This tends to appear in the areas covered by clothes i.e. body and tops of limbs, and will generally be absent from areas not covered by clothes, i.e. hands and face. Skin irritation is a form of contact dermatitis. Detergents used for washing up dishes tend to cause contact dermatitis of the hands, and especially in the webs between the fingers.

To avoid soap and detergent chemical sensitivity reduce your exposure to them by following these recommendations:

- When washing your body, use simple soap with no perfume.
- When washing clothes a non-biological detergent should be used. There are now many ecologically safe detergents on the market which are also less likely to cause allergies.
- After you have washed your clothes with powder, put them through a further washing cycle *without any powder*.

Perfumes and Cosmetics

Allergy to perfumes and cosmetics is a problem experienced almost exclusively by women. Some women are chemically sensitive both to their own and other women's perfumes and cosmetics. If you find that you are sensitive to cosmetics, then there will often be enough in the air next to a wearer to give you a problem. It is wise to use low allergy products even if you have no chemical sensitivity; however, if you do have a problem you may need to avoid them completely.

Treated Papers, Boards and Woods

Although these are all made from wood, they are impregnated with chemicals such as phenols, formaldehyde and occasionally the incredibly poisonous dioxins. Laminated boards, block boards and plywoods are a major cause of indoor pollution in modern house construction, since they give off large amounts of formaldehyde.

Chlorinated hydrocarbons (halocarbons)

The chlorine-carbon bond (Cl-C) found in chlorinated hydrocarbons has a particularly powerful effect on the immune system, stimulating it into response and often sensitivity. The chlorinated hydrocarbons are amongst the most toxic substances known. This is due to their persistence in the body fat and as 'orphan' chemicals their almost complete resistance to being broken down.

This group includes:

- organochlorine pesticides
- PCBs (polychlorinated biphenyls)
- solvents, polishes and cleaners
- plasticizers
- flame retardants
- anaesthetics and pharmaceutical drugs
- aerosol propellants (CFCs) and refrigerants

Chlorinated hydrocarbons are also produced during the chlorination of water, and bleaching of paper and many other industrial processes. PCBs are very inert substances that are excellent electric insulators but surprisingly good conductors of heat. For these properties they are used in transformers, electrical equipment and as hydraulic fluid. They can be disposed of safely only by burning at very high temperatures (greater than 1,100°C). Disposal at lower temperatures causes the creation of dioxin, a very poisonous and cancer-inducing substance.

CFCs, used as the propellant gas in aerosols, are responsible for destruction of the ozone layer.

Toxic Gases

These include carbon monoxide, oxides of nitrogen, sulphur dioxide and ozone. The first two are produced by combustion of hydrocarbons e.g. petrol, diesel, natural gas. Sulphur dioxide is the main active ingredient in acid rain, which is responsible for the destruction of forests. Sulphur dioxide and oxides of nitrogen are produced by power stations burning sulphur-containing coal. The sulphur can be removed from the exhaust gases by use of 'scrubbers'. Ozone, O_3, is produced by electrical devices, especially motors, and occurs due to poor contact and sparking. (The ozone layer surrounding the earth is not toxic because it is situated 12 to 30 miles above the earth and actually protects us against cosmic radiation.)

Toxic Metals

These include the metals, lead, mercury, cadmium and aluminium.

Lead

The main source of lead is as an antiknock agent in petrol. Lead also occurs in paint, lead pipes and joints, canned foods, juices and fruits. Fortunately, with increased green awareness and the reduced price of lead-free petrol, the amount of this poison is dropping. Another source of lead is from tins with unlined seams.

Lead is particularly destructive to children's brains. Studies have shown that high levels of lead, found in children living near motorways, cause a reduction in their IQ. Miscarriages and malformations are also more common in areas with high lead levels.

Mercury

Mercury is one of the most toxic substances known. It is particularly poisonous when combined with other molecules to form organic mercury. In Japan, it is responsible for 'Minamata disease', which is caused by the pollution of tuna fish with industrial mercury.

The commonest source of mercury pollution is dental fillings. Mercury (a liquid metal) is used to produce amalgams of gold and silver which are used for fillings. Research indicates that the mercury does not remain in the filling but is slowly leached out into the mouth from where it can be absorbed into the body. Mercury fillings have been implicated in a wide variety of diseases, including multiple sclerosis, epilepsy, psychiatric illness and ME. If amalgam fillings are removed in the correct order, i.e. the most dangerous one first, it is sometimes possible to cure these diseases. The dental cavities are, of course, refilled with a safe inert material.

Other common sources of mercury include:

- factories making paper
- polluted drinking water
- weedkillers and mercury powders used to treat seed wheat
- sea food living on the sea bed or the continental shelf
- skin lightening creams

Cadmium

The commonest source of cadmium is in cigarette smoke. However, cadmium may occur in drinking water (due to its use in plumbing alloys), evaporated milk, shellfish and paints.

Arsenic

Arsenic is found in some insecticides, wines and well waters and shellfish, and is also produced by burning coal.

Aluminium

There are several common sources of aluminium. It most frequently occurs in tap water. Aluminium salts are added as a 'fining agent' during the purification process to make biological matter such as weeds and algae drop out of suspension.

The metal enters the body from aluminium cooking pots, pans, and foil, especially when cooking acid fruits such as rhubarb, apples and leaf vegetables. Aluminium pressure cookers give an even higher dose of the metal in the food. Aluminium teapots leach the metal into solution and tea leaves have a particular ability to dissolve it. Aluminium is used to pack 'take away' foods, pre-packed frozen dinners and for some drinks cans. The metal is a component of certain foods and medicines, e.g. in coffee creamers and some indigestion mixtures.

Alcohol
Alcohols are found in plastics, cleaning products, office solvents and drugs. Alcoholic beverages e.g. spirits, wines and beer contain a particular sort of alcohol called ethyl alcohol (C_2H_5OH). However, some people who react to alcohol are, in fact, allergic to the yeast used in the fermentation, or else to the source of carbohydrate use for fermentation e.g. malted barley for whisky, grapes or other fruit for brandy, sugar cane for rum.

Ethyl alcohol drops given under the tongue can sometimes be used to desensitize a chemically sensitive patient to a wide variety of other chemicals.

Phenols
Phenol (carbolic acid) is a constituent of a very wide variety of household goods including hard plastics (Bakelite), epoxy resins, phenolic resins, synthetic detergents, carbolic soap, disinfectants, dyes, preservatives, cosmetics and deodorants, pesticides and herbicides. It also occurs in the gold-coloured lining of tin cans.

Terpenes
They are widely found in nature, especially in scented oils from pine trees and citrus fruits. Terpenes are found in the following synthetic sources: paints, motor car and gas fumes, and anaesthetics. The odour of terpenes is best described as the 'Christmas tree' smell.

Formaldehyde

Last but certainly not least, is formaldehyde. It is the single most important substance likely to induce chemical sensitivity. Approximately one person in five has a sensitivity to formaldehyde and is susceptible. It can cause symptoms at concentrations of as little as 1 part per 100 million. The symptoms are very varied, and include headaches, depression, fatigue, concentration and memory problems, dizziness, breathing problems, flushes and burnings, rashes, arthritis, flu-like illness and changes in behaviour, in other words, typical allergic symptoms.

Formaldehyde is outgassed (i.e. released as a gas), by a *very wide variety* of substances including plastics, textiles, dyes, rubbers, foams, resins, glues, papers, newsprint, disinfectants, cosmetics, soaps, shampoos, insecticides, fertilizers, chip board, block board, plywood, veneer, concrete, plaster and motor car fumes, in fact, almost every synthetic item in the modern home.

Urea formaldehyde foam insulation (UFFI) is used in modern house insulation. It is put in the cavity wall and is made by mixing two chemicals which react together to form foam, the bubbles being produced by formaldehyde. UFFI continues to release formaldehyde into the house for many years after the insulation is installed and can be a major cause of ill health. UFFI is banned in Canada. Other places which often have high formaldehyde levels include biology laboratories, shopping arcades, caravans, mobile houses and airtight houses and offices.

OUTDOOR AND INDOOR POLLUTION

It is helpful to divide chemical sensitivity into two groups on the basis of the source of pollution causing the problem.

- Outdoor pollution
- Indoor pollution

The two usually have completely different causes. Although the treatment in both cases is avoidance, this is achieved in different ways.

Superficially, it would appear that outdoor pollution is a more serious problem than indoor pollution. However, in practice, the opposite is the case. Indoor pollution causes chemical sensitivity in 8 to 10 times as many people as outdoor pollution. This is why your chemical sensitivity is likely to be better outdoors, and in the summer, and worse indoors and in the winter when ventilation is reduced and the central heating is on. (This is, clearly, completely the opposite pattern to hayfever which is worse outdoors in summer and better indoors in winter).

OUTDOOR POLLUTION

Outdoor pollution causing chemical sensitivity is usually intermittent rather than continuous. It can be predicted by the following factors:

- The amount of neotoxin released by the source, e.g. factory chimney, car fumes from underpasses, pesticide spray.
- How close you are to the source of neotoxins (for the technically minded, the amount of neotoxin you receive is usually proportional to the inverse square of the distance from the source).
- The amount of time that you are exposed to the neotoxin. If you are sensitive to sulphur dioxide from a factory chimney, you may be able to drive past the factory without symptoms. However, if you live or work near the factory, then you will be constantly unwell.

The above three factors can be expressed in the formula which applies to all neotoxins, (biological, chemical, physical and mental):

$$\text{Dose of neotoxin} = \text{Amount of neotoxin} \times \text{Proximity to source of neotoxin} \times \text{Time exposed to neotoxin}$$

Other factors influencing reaction to outdoor pollutants are:

- The wind direction. Any location which is within 50 miles downwind of a large city is likely to suffer pollution. The wind usually blows from one direction, (the prevailing wind), which means the areas downwind in the direction of the prevailing wind will be worst affected, whereas other areas will tend to be spared.
- The wind strength. Static air and winds above 15 miles per hour reduce the likelihood of chemical sensitivity, whereas mild breezes increase the risk.
- The humidity and cloud cover. The more humid the atmosphere, the more likely that an airborne chemical will induce a chemical sensitivity. The most obvious example of this is fog, which when mixed with a chemical pollutant becomes smog. Exposure to smog for a day or two can induce a permanent sensitivity which will affect you for the rest of your life.
- Geography of an area. Some areas, e.g. Los Angeles, being located in a natural bowl-shaped area, tend to trap pollutants which then linger.

One useful way to assess the level of outdoor pollution is by measuring visibility. As a general rule, the greater the distance you can see, the less the level of outdoor pollution.

INDOOR POLLUTION

- Modern construction methods
  This involves the use of materials that outgas formaldehyde and other organic fumes. These materials include chip board, block board, particle board, treated timbers and plywood, plastics, solvents, glues, paints and varnishes, pesticides and fungicides.
- Modern furnishing methods
  Extensive use of man made fabrics, carpets and plastics produces a large 'load' of formaldehyde and other gases.

- Lack of ventilation
  Many modern buildings have airtight seals on the windows and are designed to have little or no outside ventilation. In large buildings, air conditioning and ventilation systems recirculate indoor air without removing the formaldehyde and other gases. Consequently, the air 'purification' system tends to concentrate gases that may induce chemical sensitivities.
- The heating system/kitchen
  These may be the origin of fumes that induce chemical sensitivity.
- Wide use of cleaners, polishes, solvents, aerosols, air fresheners and disinfectants
- Integral garages and storerooms
  These allow vehicle combustion fumes and other solvent fumes to enter working and living areas.
- Wide use of plastic-covered electronic devices
  Apart from the electric and magnetic fields which are physical neotoxins, these cause problems because they get hot and release chemical fumes and ozone, e.g. television sets, photocopying machines, and power tools.
- Biological neotoxins
  These are not chemical neotoxins. However, they contribute to the total load of neotoxins in the house. They are dealt with elsewhere in the book.

HOW DO I FIND OUT TO WHICH CHEMICALS I AM SENSITIVE?

This is similar to the methods used for food allergy testing. It involves excluding chemical neotoxins from your body, as far as possible, and then 'challenging' yourself with suspected substances. This is a specialized process and should be carried out by an experienced practitioner of Environmental Medicine.

The following chapter will help you to reduce your load of chemical as well as other neotoxins.

12

Hayfever Treatment Plan

The hayfever plan is likely to reduce the number and severity of your hayfever symptoms but, failing that, it is very likely to improve your general health.

You will need to review your present lifestyle, identifying the activities, places and times when you may be suffering from neotoxins. Then you can change your lifestyle so that you get rid of the acquired problem. You can do this by following the three rules:

1) reduce your total load of neotoxins.
2) reduce particularly the neotoxin(s) to which you are especially sensitive.
3) use sleep, rest, exercise, vitamins, minerals and other supplements to help yourself back to complete health.

If you have read the first part of the book, you have probably started thinking about which neotoxins affect you, by working out which kind of pollen may be causing your hayfever. Now that you have read chapters 10 and 11, it is time to think carefully about which other types of neotoxins you may be exposed to (also see below) and make a list of them. Try to decide which activity, place, and time makes your allergic symptoms better or worse. For example, are your symptoms worse on Monday morning when you return to work after the weekend? Do they improve when you visit a friend's house? These include not only symptoms of hayfever, but also the symptoms listed on page 123 or any of those on page 75.

It is helpful to split the day into thirds when you are making your list. Think about your load of neotoxins separately at:

work ⎫ Each takes approximately
home and hobbies ⎬ 8 hours
sleep, bedroom ⎭ of your day

You may well have your suspicions about which neotoxins are affecting you. *Superhealth*, by the same author, contains detailed questionnaires which help you to assess your lifestyle and your exposure to neotoxins.

You will need to follow the relevant chapters (chapter 10 on food and biological neotoxins and chapter 11 on chemical neotoxins) to decide an individual susceptibility, but the rest of this chapter will tell you how to reduce your total load of neotoxins.

REDUCING THE TOTAL LOAD OF BIOLOGICAL NEOTOXINS

Organic Food
Eat only organic food (i.e. nothing that has been sprayed with chemicals or pesticides). You can be happy that it is organic if it has the imprint of the Soil Association. Try to avoid anything from a packet, tin or bottle, especially if it contains any additives (E numbers).

Bottled Water
Drink and cook with bottled water only, preferably from glass bottles. Drink at least 3 pints of fluid a day as this will help to flush out poisons from your body.

Food Preparation
Prepare your food properly and be careful not to handle cooked and uncooked meats with the same utensils. Cook thoroughly and avoid the use of microwave ovens.

Pets and Indoor Pollens
If you are allergic to your pets or flowers, try to keep them out of the house as much as possible. Even if you are not allergic, make sure you keep pets and flowers out of your bedroom (you sleep in there for about 8 hours).

Outdoor Pollens
If you have hayfever, keep your windows closed during the day in the hayfever season. You may open them briefly after heavy rainstorms, when pollen levels are greatly reduced.

Damp and Fungi
Keep your house dry, especially your bedroom. Damp encourages growth of fungi and house dust mites.

House Dust Mite
If you are allergic to house dust mites (i.e. you suffer from rhinitis, runny eyes or asthma which is worse in bed), then follow the measures described on page 59 to remove house dust mite.

Infections
Take all reasonable steps to avoid all sources of infections.

REDUCING THE TOTAL LOAD OF CHEMICAL NEOTOXINS

Reduce your total load of chemical neotoxins at home by the following methods:

Correct Site for Your House
People allergic to trees or grass pollens should avoid woods and fields. Then find the direction of the prevailing wind. Avoid being near or downwind of industrial areas, factories, chemical dumps, busy roads, especially junctions, or agricultural land that is sprayed. A house site needs to be well drained to avoid damp which causes the growth of fungi. Don't live in a house built on a landfill

site, since these outgas methane, or else highly toxic chemicals may have been dumped there.

Construction
Modern house construction methods release a very wide range of chemicals. Urea Formaldehyde Foam Insulation (UFFI) in cavity walls is now banned in Canada. Any house with this form of insulation is totally unsatisfactory, since the UFFI continues to release formaldehyde into the house for years after the installation. Wide use of formaldehyde-releasing woods, boards, plastics, glues and paints is also unacceptable. Asbestos should also be avoided since it raises the risk of cancer. Recent spraying with antifungals (e.g. pentachlorophenol) is also very dangerous.

Furnishings and Decorations
Remove as many synthetic fabrics, foams, carpets, curtains, plywood, block board and plastics as possible. Replace these with metal, glass, unbleached natural fibres and bare wood or tiles.

Heating
Review the heating system of the house. Try to replace natural gas with electricity (unless you are electrically sensitive). If you have a boiler, try to have it sited in a sealed room which does not communicate with the rest of the house. Make sure the chimneys and flues remove the exhaust gases fully so that they do not leak back into the house.

Cooking
Consider changing your natural gas cooker to an electric one. If you decide to change your gas cooker, you should also have all the old gas pipes removed. Unused gas pipes will still continue to leak tiny amounts of gas. Replace your teflon and aluminium cooking utensils with glass and stainless steel.

Ventilation
Increase the ventilation through the house, especially in the kitchen and bedroom, by installing extractor fans.

Clothing

Wear only natural unbleached fibres coloured with natural dyes. Try to make sure that fibres have not been treated with pesticides for moth proofing.

Aerosols and Beauty Products

Completely avoid aerosols since the propellants are the highly allergic fluorinated hydrocarbons (CFCs). Also try to avoid using cosmetics, deodorants and other beauty products since they often cause problems.

Washing

When washing your body, use only plain soap without perfume. When washing your clothes use a non-biological detergent. After washing, rinse your clothes with an extra washing cycle without powder.

Storage

Don't store bleaches, cleaners, disinfectants and polishes in parts of the house that you frequently use. Also start using less chemically active substances for these purposes. Fortunately the Green movement is providing alternatives which are much less toxic to the environment and similarly to humans. It is not necessary to 'kill all known germs' so use these materials very sparingly.

Garage

If you have an integral garage, don't park your car in there because fumes will come into the house, and especially into the room above the garage.

Smoking

Give up smoking. If you don't smoke but somebody else in the house is a smoker, do your best to persuade them not to smoke indoors. Otherwise, try to get them to restrict their smoking to rooms that you don't use.

Sleeping
You spend 8 hours a day in your bedroom. However, unfortunately, the average bedroom is filled with many possible sources of chemical sensitivity. Even if you don't change any other part of your house, convert your bedroom to a chemically clean area. Consider using a small room for a bedroom, and adapt it as follows:

First move everything non-essential out.
Remove all the synthetic fabrics, foams, carpets and plastics, and replace them with non-bleached cotton and wool bedding and metal and glass fittings.
Try to store your clothes, books and other possessions somewhere else, since they tend to give off formaldehyde.

Chemical Neotoxins in the Office
Reduce your total load of chemical neotoxins by the following methods:

Choice of Office
If you have the choice, avoid a modern air conditioned office with no opening windows. These frequently cause illnesses such as the 'Sick Building Syndrome'.

Avoid Solvents
Try to avoid all solvents. Stop using marker pens, liquid typewriter correcting fluid and glues.

Photocopying Machines
Try to make sure that the photocopying machine is located in a well ventilated spot away from the work area.

Avoid Polishes and Cleaners
Try to avoid excessive use of polishes, waxes, carpet cleaners, air fresheners, antiseptics and fly and insect sprays.

No Smoking
Encourage the office to have a no smoking policy.

Turn Off Electrical Devices

Turn off all electrical devices when they are not in use. These give off many fumes and in addition, an increasing number of people are electrically sensitive.

Chemical Neotoxins in the Factory

Reduce your total load of chemical neotoxins in your factory by the following methods:

Protective Clothing

Wear all the protective clothing provided for the job. The Health and Safety Executive is a UK government body with wide powers and can advise on current safety equipment **which must be provided for your use by law.**

However, chemical sensitivities occur at concentrations of chemicals far below the present 'safe' level. If you are chemically sensitive, then you may decide to find alternative employment rather than continually making yourself ill.

Activated Carbon Filter Mask

Wear an activated carbon filter mask. This will extract a large number of chemical neotoxins from the air that you breathe. This mask must fit tightly and must be renewed regularly.

Ventilation

Ensure that there is good ventilation of fresh clean air in your work area. Check all flues, chimneys and air ducts.

Avoid Solvents

Use all volatile and airborne substances, e.g. solvents, paints, glues, either outdoors or in special areas designed for their use. Wear protective masks.

No Smoking

Do not smoke. Encourage the factory to have a no-smoking policy.

REDUCING THE TOTAL LOAD OF PHYSICAL NEOTOXINS

Reduce your total load of physical neotoxins by these methods:

Avoid EM Radiation
Try not to live or work near a high voltage power line, electric motor, generator or transformer, transmitter, nuclear reactor or reprocessing plant, or military installations.

Reduce Exposure to VDUs
Reduce your exposure to electric and magnetic fields by turning off all devices when not in use, e.g. turn off VDUs and don't use them for more than 4 hours a day, or more than an a hour at a time without a break.

High Risk Electrical Devices
Completely avoid using electric overblankets, heated water beds, sunbeds and microwave ovens.

X-rays and Conception
Don't have any unnecessary x-ray investigations, especially in the 3 months before you plan to conceive a child. This rule applies to men as well as women.

Reduce Noise Level
Reduce your work and home sound level so that you can easily hold a conversation in a normal speaking voice.

REDUCING THE TOTAL LOAD OF MENTAL NEOTOXINS

Reduce your total load of mental neotoxins by these methods:

Have Reasonable Objectives
Decide on a very few well defined reasonable objectives and don't take on too many tasks.

Have a Positive Response to Stress

Change your response to stress. Always try to be positive and constructive, but also learn from your mistakes. Don't worry too much. One of the best ways to do this is to see life as a game in which sometimes you win and sometimes you lose.

Use Relaxation Techniques

Use relaxation techniques to cope with stress. Make sure that you get enough daily exercise and sleep. Natural relaxation and sex are also very helpful as is a strong relationship with another person.

No Instant Solution

Avoid 'instant' 20th century remedies to produce relaxation such as tranquillizers, TV, cigarettes and alcohol. There are no short cuts!

Have the Right Mental Attitude

By far the most important single factor stopping you from getting better from almost anything is not having the right mental attitude. The right mental attitude is on the one hand an acceptance that you have a health problem, followed on the other by a willingness to do whatever is necessary in order to beat the problem. Without this positive attitude any therapy or treatment is likely to be less effective.

Have the Right Plan

Sometimes the problem is not so much that you don't try hard, but rather that you're working at the wrong things. It is very easy to be frantically busy, bailing out a sinking ship, rather than taking time out in order to decide how to plug the leaks once and for all. After all, when you've stopped the water gushing in, it's relatively easy to bail out the boat at your leisure.

EXERCISE

The modern 20th century lifestyle actually makes it quite difficult to exercise. Insufficient attention and resources are devoted to helping people to make exercise part of their lives. Exercise for adults is often seen as a television spectator sport.

Your plan to treat your hayfever needs to include physical exercise and mental relaxation. You can do this in two ways:

by identifying changes that you can make in your lifestyle so that you are able to increase the exercise content of your day with only a little extra effort;
by planning a thirty minute vigorous session twice or three times a week at an activity you enjoy.

A personal fitness plan is not a new idea, and in fact it was quite usual for the ancient Greeks to consult both a physician and a trainer in order to recover from illness. The former would diagnose and treat ailments, and the latter would work out a customized series of exercises and activities to get the patient back to fitness and health.

Exercise Tips

- Don't ride when you can walk.
- Park your car, or get off the bus several stops before your destination, and walk the remaining distance.
- Change your route so you can walk or run through the park (in daylight) on the way to work.
- Use the stairs, not the lift. If it is a multi-storey building, get out four floors before your destination and walk the last four floors (your colleagues will be very impressed). If you are feeling a little less energetic, go four floors above your destination and walk down: it is still exercise. Do the same when leaving.
- Don't do everything by telephone. Make a personal visit sometimes. The exercise and face-to-face contact will help you work more efficiently.
- Buy a bicycle to ride to work. However, don't ride it in smog-filled underpasses or in the rain or snow, when cycling is often dangerous.

- Use exercise as a substitute for other things you are cutting out of your life, such as cigarettes, alcohol, food.
- Use exercise as part of your stress management programme.

VITAMINS AND MINERAL DEFICIENCIES

Adequate amounts of vitamins, minerals and other nutrients are essential for good health. They are particularly important in allergic disease, since they help the body to repair itself. During an allergic illness the daily requirement of a specific vitamin, mineral or other nutrient may be dramatically increased.

Deficiencies of vitamins, minerals and other nutrients may occur because of the following reasons:

Inadequate Dietary Intake for the State of Health
Allergic and ill people need more vitamins and minerals. The Recommended Daily Allowance (RDA) which is so often quoted is the minimum amount needed by fit people to stop deficiency disease. This is not a meaningful figure, since the amount required for *optimum* health is usually considerably higher, especially in an ill person.

Interaction of Vitamins and Minerals with Other Substances and Bacteria in the Gut
Despite having an adequate dietary intake, a deficiency may arise due to interaction of vitamins and minerals with other substances found in the gut (e.g. vitamin D being bound to phytic acid in flour). The bacteria normally living in the bowel can be altered after a course of antibiotics and then the altered bacteria may destroy vitamins.

Failure of Absorption
If the bowel is damaged physically or biochemically it is unable to absorb vitamins and minerals properly. Physical damage occurs in coeliac disease when the convoluted (and consequently high

surface area) small bowel is replaced with a flat (and much lower surface area) bowel. Biochemical damage occurs after infection or poisoning, at which time enzyme damage occurs active absorption is greatly reduced.

Failure of Utilization
After vitamins and minerals are absorbed, they enter the circulation. However, sometimes they cannot be used properly due to a deficiency of another substance. For example, this failure of utilization may occur when adequate levels of Vitamin B_{12} cannot be used unless folic acid is also present in adequate amounts.

HOW CAN I ENSURE THAT I GET ADEQUATE VITAMINS AND MINERALS?

- Have a varied diet: don't eat the same thing every day. Instead rotate food families (see page 112), and occasionally stop eating a popular food for three days.
- Buy fresh food and eat soon after purchase. Vitamin content is reduced by light, and storage at room temperature. Refrigeration, cooling and dark reduce the rate of vitamin lost.
- Where possible, cook and eat fruit and vegetables with the skin on, as the vitamin content is much higher. Try to use organic fruit and vegetables, as chemicals penetrate sprayed fruit and high levels of poison may be absorbed, particularly if the skin is eaten.
- When preparing and cooking food, avoid prolonged soaking or cooking because this reduces vitamin content.
- Cook your food in bottled water. Tap water often contains unacceptable contaminants.
- Eat food immediately after cooking. Standing reduces vitamin content. Vitamins and mineral deficiencies are quite common in the Western World due to:
    low vitamin and mineral content of food
    the increased requirements secondary to stress, pollution and allergies.

Most people need vitamin and mineral supplements. The exact dose should be tailored to your individual requirements, e.g. for children, men, women (pregnant, breast feeding), in sickness or in health.

It is important to remember that although the body is able to synthesize some of the vitamins, it cannot make any mineral. Consequently, it is essential that these are taken either in the diet or as a supplement.

Some general guidelines for adults are given table 12.1.

Table 12.1: Suggested Daily Vitamin Supplement for Adults

A	5,000 iu	
B$_1$	50 mg ⎫	B Complex vitamins
B$_2$	50 mg ⎪	The 'anti-stress' vitamins
B$_3$	100 mg ⎬	should be taken together
B$_5$	100 mg ⎪	rather than singly
B$_6$	100 mg ⎭	
C	2,000 mg	The 'anti-pollution' vitamin
E	200 iu	The 'antioxidant' vitamin
Calcium	500 mg	Take as Dolomite tablet
Magnesium	250 mg	The 'anti-stress' mineral. Take as Dolomite tablet
Zinc	15 mg	Take as chelated zinc if possible
Evening Primrose Oil	1,500 mg	Source of essential Omega 6 fatty acids

NB: The daily dosage of vitamins and minerals will need to be increased during pregnancy and breast-feeding. The doses for children are considerably less than the adult dose. Ideally, vitamin intake should be supervised by a suitably qualified practitioner and tailored to each individual's requirements.

When you are taking vitamins and minerals, try to follow these guidelines:

• Make sure there are no additives, colours or flavours in the mineral or vitamin supplement. Check that you are not allergic to the filler, e.g. lactose (milk sugar) or cornflour which makes up the bulk of the tablet.

- Take *chelated* mineral tablets if available. A chelated mineral is more easily absorbed. Non-chelated minerals are less well absorbed, especially in ill patients, and the dose received is far less.
- Vitamins and minerals reduce the effectiveness of antibiotics. If you are taking antibiotics, take your supplement one hour before or two hours after the antibiotic.
- Take vitamins that come from natural sources rather than synthetically produced ones. Although the vitamins from both sources are chemically identical, the other substances found with the naturally occurring vitamins make it more effective and less likely to cause side effects.

How Can I Tell if I Have a Vitamin or Mineral Deficiency?
Unfortunately, there is no easy way to tell if you have a vitamin or mineral deficiency. There are recognized vitamin deficiency symptoms, but many of these have a gradual onset and are very similar to allergic symptoms. If you take the vitamin supplements as advised, you are much less likely to be deficient.

Mineral deficiencies in contrast, can be confirmed by carrying out a hair analysis. It is essential to have your results interpreted by an expert to understand the full significance of the test. The technique of hair analysis is also able to show the presence of toxic metals such as mercury, aluminium, arsenic and cadmium.

13

Alternative Treatments

It's not just a bad pun to say that alternative or complementary medicine has a field day with hayfever. The effects of the pollen sensitivity often can be greatly reduced, if not cured by therapies such as:

- Nutritional therapy (see chapter 10)
- Chemical detoxification (see chapter 11)
- Homoeopathy (see p 160)
- Provocation/neutralization and isopathy (see p 165)
- Schüssler tissue salts (see p 166)
- Bach flower remedies (see p 166)
- Acupuncture (see p 167)
- Reflex therapy (see p 168)
- Aromatherapy (see p 169)
- Herbal medicine (see p 169).

Many patients already benefiting from one or more of these therapies will realize that, in order to get the best results, it is essential to attend a fully-qualified practitioner who works holistically. You will receive the best treatment from the most experienced practitioner who looks at all your circumstances and works out a treatment plan specific to your personality, temperament and situation in life.

In general, you get less success if you use alternative or complementary forms of medicine for merely treating isolated symptoms such as hayfever. However, as with most things in life, there are qualified exceptions. Homoeopathy may be used for what is known as 'first-aid' prescribing, in which the symptoms are matched with a remedy that has a similar symptom picture (see table 13.1). In 'first-aid' prescribing, what are known as 'low potencies', like the 6c potency, are used and repeated frequently. These low potencies have a 'superficial' effect on physical symptoms, unlike high potencies (e.g. the 200C, MC and 10MC potencies) which have a much more profound effect on all systems. High potencies are used for 'constitutional' prescribing in which the remedy selected is a precise match to the patient's personality, temperament and total symptom picture.

The aim here is to give you a working introduction to homoeopathy, which you can then use for 'first-aid' prescribing for yourself and your family. One of the great advantages of homoeopathy is that, unlike conventional drugs, low potencies of homoeopathic remedies very rarely give side effects. Even if you have selected the wrong homoeopathic remedy, you are unlikely to become ill as a side effect of the treatment. Also in this chapter there are brief introductory sections about other alternative therapies which are useful in the treatment of hayfever, to give you some idea of the likely benefits of attending the appropriate practitioner.

WHAT IS HOMOEOPATHY?

Homoeopathy is an alternative medicine started 200 years ago by Dr Samuel Hahnemann, a German physician.

There are three basic principles:

Like Cures Like
Hence the term *homoeopathy* (Greek: *homoios* - similar; *pathos* - disease). In other words, if a substance causes an illness, or symptoms similar to that illness in a healthy person, then that substance can be used to treat the illness.

For example, the poison white arsenic when given in a high dose produces burning in the eyes, a thin watery discharge, and a burning throat. These are very similar to the symptoms of hayfever. Thus, if used homoeopathically, white arsenic (Arsen Alb) may be employed to treat hayfever.

The More Dilute the Substance, the Greater its Potency
Potency = the ability of the substance to cure disease.
This is quite the opposite to the usual experience in life. If you want a detergent or bleach to work better, then it is used undiluted. However, the above law is based on the observation that in biological systems a high dose of a substance, e.g. strychnine, may poison but a low dose may stimulate, as in strychnine nerve tonic.

Homoeopathy Treats the Whole Person, Not Just the Disease
In order to find the most suitable homoeopathic remedy, apart from first-aid prescribing, all the patient's symptoms must be considered and precisely defined. For example, in the case of a chest problem does the patient have a dry cough, a productive cough, is it better for heat or cold, is it better or worse at night, is there an associated headache, and so on. Also, many other factors at present ignored by conventional medicine must be considered, e.g. personality, temperament, body build, age, sex, hair colour etc. Conventional medicine treats only organs, not the whole person, and gives to everyone the same drug for an illness, irrelevant of the factors considered above - e.g. penicillin is nearly always given for a chest infection. Homoeopathy gives many different remedies for the same medical diagnosis according to the needs to each individual and their specific symptoms.

HOW ARE HOMOEOPATHIC REMEDIES PRODUCED?

Any substance can be prepared homoeopathically but the usual classification of remedy sources is animal, vegetable, mineral, chemical, drugs and products of disease (known as nosodes).

The method of preparation is similar in all cases, although there may be slight variations to take account of solubility in alcohol of the source material. The commonest method involves making an alcoholic extract of the material in question, such as white arsenic to make Arsen Alb. This alcoholic extract is the most concentrated solution of the substance that can be made. It is termed the Mother Tincture. This is then diluted many times over with an alcohol/water mixture. The sixth centesimal potency, or 6c, means one drop of mother tincture to 1,000,000,000,000 of the diluting mixture. (This dilution is roughly comparable to one drop of mother tincture in the combined volume of 50 Olympic-sized swimming pools.) This final dilution is added to lactose tablets which then become 'potentized'.

WHY DOES HOMOEOPATHY WORK?

Scientifically speaking, at any potency past 12c the remedy is so dilute that there should not be any molecules of the original substance present in the homoeopathic remedy. This emphasizes the fact that homoeopathy does not work by the conventional laws of drug action, but rather the incredibly minute doses of the right remedy stimulate the body and restore vital energy. This restoration of vital energy is a thread that runs through almost all forms of alternative medicine.

The ideal homoeopathic remedy consists of a single dose of a single remedy which is tailored to suit the patient. The ideal remedy then works very quickly and with very few side effects or interactions with other drugs. Unlike conventional medicines, which appear to work by suppressing symptoms and eventually suppressing the body's own powers of healing, homoeopathic medicines stimulate the body's power to heal itself. If an illness is merely suppressed and not cured it is possible that the disease process will move inward, towards more vital organs, and upwards (e.g. when eczema of the skin is suppressed with steroid creams, asthma may arise).

TAKING THE REMEDY

If the correct remedy is given, then there is often an *initial aggravation* of the symptoms, followed by an improvement. In addition, it has been found that healing occurs in the reverse order of development of symptoms, the first symptoms to appear being the last to disappear and vice versa. Also, the cure starts with

the inner and most important organs, moving outwards
   and
the upper parts of the body, moving downwards to lower parts.

The longer that a symptom, or disease, has been present, the longer it takes for a homoeopathic medicine to produce a cure. The minimum possible dose should be used and the more accurately that the remedy fits the illness, the smaller the dose that will be required. The remedy should be stopped as soon as an improvement commences and should not be repeated so long as it continues to act. Usually, there will be an improvement within two weeks of starting a remedy, provided that it is correct but, if there is no improvement in one month, then a different remedy should be considered.

The earlier that a homoeopathic remedy is given after the onset of an illness, the better. The patient should be treated as soon as symptoms appear and *before* there is actual physical damage to the organs or tissues. If the illness is caught early, often the disease-induced changes can be fully reversed, leaving no permanent problem.

Do not handle the homoeopathic preparations. Tip the tablet(s) into the lid and drop straight into the mouth. The homoeopathic medicine should not be swallowed but chewed or sucked. The medicine is directly absorbed from the mouth and, provided the correct remedy has been chosen, works almost instantaneously. The medicine should be taken without water and put into a 'clean mouth', i.e. free of food, drink (especially alcohol and coffee), tobacco, toothpaste and sweets.

Always store the medicines in the bottle prescribed, away from light and strong-smelling substances, e.g. antiseptics, aftershave, perfume, toothpaste, menthol or camphor. Do not store in a bathroom cabinet, in other words.

WHAT REMEDIES ARE USEFUL TO TREAT HAYFEVER?

The following tables show remedies that are useful for hayfever.

The way to decide which remedy is most able to help you is to match your symptom picture with that of the remedy. Once you have found a remedy that works well for you, keep a note of the name.

Homoeopathic remedies useful before before hayfever season starts, as well as during season.

Remedy	Eye symptoms	Nasal symptoms	Ear/throat/chest	Other comments
ARSEN ALB	Burning hot eyes with dislike of light	Thin watery burning discharge	Offensive discharge	Very
ARUNDO		Annoying itching of nostrils/ sneezing	Itching roof of mouth	Useful for Catarrh
CHROM ALUM	Red swollen eyelids, with tears	sneezing		
WYETHIA		Itching at the back of nostrils	Throat swollen Dry hacking cough	Useful for throat

Useful hayfever remedies for use during season

Remedy	Eye symptoms	Nasal symptoms	Ear/throat/ chest	Other comments
ALLIUM CEPA	Burning eyes, Smarting eyes Dislike of light		Hacking cough, tickling in throat	Compare to the effect of peeling onions
EUPHROLIA	Constantly watering eyes		Violent cough, with much expectoration	
GELSEMIUM	Painful heavy eyelids	Watery discharge	Lump in throat with sneezing	
NATRUM MUR	Bruised eyes	Sneezing violently with watery discharge		
	Sabadilla	Burning red eyelids	Intermittent sneezing with runny norse	Sore throat better after warm drink

ISOPATHY AND PROVOCATION/NEUTRALIZATION

Homoeopathy works by giving the patient a substance that, if used by a healthy person, would produce a similar symptom picture to the one that the patient is experiencing. If, however, it is known which substance (e.g. birch pollen) is causing the symptoms, then it is possible to prepare homoeopathically an extract of birch pollen, which in many cases has an effect of 'desensitizing' the patient to that substance. Strictly speaking this is not homoeopathy but *isopathy*. Homoeopathically prepared extracts of trees, grasses, weeds, fungi and animal fur are all available from homoeopathic suppliers.

Provocation/neutralization testing and treatment uses a method that is basically similar to isopathy, although many more dilutions are used. Each dilution is 1/5th the strength of the previous dilution. The provocation neutralization is carried out either by injecting the extract under the skin, or else by putting drops of the diluted solution into the mouth and looking for the appearance and disappearance of symptoms. Although it is unclear how this works, in many allergic patients one dilution often provokes symptoms, but a second more dilute solution neutralizes those symptoms. The skill is to find the neutralizing point strength for all the important substances causing problems and then make these up into a mixture to treat the symptoms.

SCHÜSSLER TISSUE SALTS

This is an alternative system of medical treatment, combining homoeopathy and a way of correcting disturbances in body minerals. The technique was devised by Dr W. Schüssler, who worked out a system to correct these disturbances by using his 12 tissue salts or vital minerals, also known as biochemic tissue salts. The remedies are potentized at the 6x level and are easily available at health food shops. Table 13.2 suggests some of the more useful remedies available for hayfever. These remedies are taken four times a day (adults 4 tablets, children 2 tablets). The best results are obtained by starting treatment several months before the start of the hayfever season.

BACH FLOWER REMEDIES

When considering hayfever it is rather appropriate that there is a whole branch of alternative/complementary medicine based on

Table 13.2: Tissue salts useful for hayfever

Name of remedy	Indication for use and comments
Ferrum Phos	Red, burning and congested eyes and nose. Headache
Kali Mur	Large amount of thin watery discharge running from eyes and nose. Also irritation and sneezing
Kali Phos	Thick catarrh produced by eyes and nose. Swelling of glands. Dry cough and asthma

flowers. However, Bach flower remedies have their greatest effect on mental symptoms and emotional states such as anger, fear, grief and impatience. These remedies are based on essences of 38 different species of wild flowers that have been prepared by soaking in pure water illuminated by bright sunlight. The concentrated remedy is then diluted before being taken as drops when required. As with many forms of alternative medicine, Bach remedies are trying to restore the body's vital energy, but the remedy must be tailored to the individual. Table 13.3 gives some of the Bach flower remedies that have been found to be helpful in hayfever together with the personality for which each is most appropriate. One of the best ways to gain confidence in the Bach flower remedies is to keep Rescue Remedy (which is a combination of 5 flowers) in your handbag or a drawer. Use it immediately after a shock or accident.

The Bach flower remedies are available from health food shops but also direct from the Bach Centre, Wallingford, nr. Oxford.

ACUPUNCTURE

Acupuncture is part of a complete system of medicine which has been developed in China over the past 5,000 years. The theory is that in the normal body 'energy' needs to flow along channels called meridians between major organs in order to maintain health. Illness occurs when this energy flow is blocked at one or more

Table 13.3: Bach Flower Remedies

Name of remedy	Personality Type Suited
Centaury	Timid, low vitality with little drive to heal self
Clematis	Withdrawn, listless, poor concentration
Crab apple	Concerned with feelings of uncleanliness
Gorse	Material and physical despair and extreme hopelessness
Star of Bethlehem	Grief, sadness, shock, numbness
Walnut	Frustration, dissatisfaction
Wild rose	Exhaustion, apathy, resignation

points. Empirically, it has been found that this energy flow can be restored by stimulating the appropriate points on these meridians, either by inserting very fine acupuncture needles and/or by the burning of herbs (moxibustion) at these points.

Traditional Chinese acupuncture is particularly useful for treating mental and psychological symptoms. Providing that acupuncture is used in a holistic way, a high degree of success can usually be expected. It is wise to avoid inexperienced acupuncturists who merely treat hayfever symptoms, rather than looking at the whole picture. The Institute for Complementary Medicine can help you to obtain a list of qualified practitioners.

REFLEXOLOGY OR REFLEX THERAPY

Reflexology works on the principle that the body can be divided into different 'reflex zones' and that 'maps' of these, representing the complete human anatomy, occur on the underside of the foot and other parts of the body.

An experienced reflex therapist can find changes at points on the foot which represent diseased organs or systems of your body, or just areas of local tension. By appropriate use of stimulation by massage and pressure, it is possible to heal a diseased organ through an effect similar to acupuncture. Although several of these 'maps' of the body can be found, the most common area used for treatment by reflex therapists are the feet. As with the other therapies, by far the best results are obtained by visiting an experienced practitioner who works holistically.

AROMATHERAPY

This is a very old medical art which can be traced back as far as ancient Egypt. It uses 'essential oils' from plants, which are prepared using flowers, leaves and seeds, roots and bark. The oils work due to both their stimulating effect on the skin when massaged in at the appropriate points, and also by inhalation. By far the best results are obtained when attending experienced, qualified practitioners who practice holistically. Table 13.4 gives a very brief introduction to 'first aid' use of aromatherapy oils.

Table 13.4: Aromatherapy oils useful for hayfever

Name of oils	Indication for use and comments
Balm	Acts as a defensive shield to combat stress, anxiety, depression and allergies
Chamomile	Acts in an anti-inflammatory and soothing way
Eucalyptus	Acts as an antiseptic, anti-inflammatory and decongestant. It stimulates and refreshes
Lavender	Acts as an antiseptic and anti-inflammatory. Soothes stress, anxiety and depression
Rose	Acts as an antiseptic, healing oil, very mild and useful for balancing body energies

HERBAL MEDICINE

Herbal Medicine is based on remedies, prepared from plants, that have been handed down over the years. Herbal preparations can be just as efficacious as pharmaceutical drugs, but the whole plant is used rather than the single chemical which is often extracted from plants to make pharmaceutical drugs.

Best results are obtained by consulting a experienced and fully qualified herbalist or naturopath, who will look at your complete symptom picture. There are some herbs that may be used in a 'first aid' fashion (see table 13.5).

Table 13.5: Herbs that may help in hayfever

Name of Herb	Indication for Use and Comments
Coltsfoot	Very useful for chest symptoms. Soothes and clears throat and chest
Echinacea	A widely-used herb to clear infections. Works by boosting immune system. Take prophylactically from March
Eyebright	First time treatment for hayfever. Either take internally or as dilute solution locally to eyes
Garlic	Helps body to clear thick secretions. A useful herb to use with echinacea
Golden rod	Helps to dry mucous membranes and stop excessive secretions and sneezing
Mullein	Similar action to golden rod
Red sage	Useful for sore throat and mouth

14

Hayfever and Your Child; Hayfever and Exams

Prevention is always better than cure. This chapter will tell you ways in which you can reduce the likelihood of your child suffering from hayfever and also many other allergic diseases.

HOW CAN I STOP MY CHILD FROM DEVELOPING HAYFEVER?

There are four different stages at which you can reduce your child's risk of suffering from hayfever. These are:

- preconception
- during pregnancy
- infancy
- early childhood to teens

As a general rule, the earlier you spot a lifestyle mistake, the less damage it does. Consequently, the best time to stop your child from getting hayfever is not just before the child is born but before the child is even conceived.

PRECONCEPTUAL CARE

The principle behind preconceptual care is to take antenatal care one vital stage further. It is an excellent way to improve your fertility and reduce your child's risk of malformation and future allergy. As a general rule, the healthier the parents, the healthier the offspring. If one or both parents suffer from illness, especially allergic disease, it is particularly important for them to change their lifestyle so that they are in peak health for the six months before conception. Preconceptual measures need to be started this early because the first three months are necessary to get rid of neotoxins and to correct vitamin and mineral deficiencies in both partners. During the second three-month period, the male can start to produce the best quality sperm that he is capable of, which has the least chance of passing on a congenital weakness, like susceptibility to hayfever. The female is most likely to pass on hereditary problems if she is exposed to adverse environmental factors in the month before conception, followed by the nine months of pregnancy.

The time of year of birth also has an important effect on the risk of developing hayfever. Many doctors were initially scornful of this finding; however, the mechanism is fairly straightforward. A child is most vulnerable to developing an allergy like hayfever when exposed to pollen aged between three and six months. The baby has a 'honeymoon' period, in which allergy is unlikely to develop, in the first three months after birth. This is because antibodies which have travelled through the placenta from the mother are still in circulation within the baby's body. They decline to negligible levels at about six months. To a lesser extent breast-fed children are being topped up with mother's antibodies, which explains why breast-fed babies have a lower incidence of allergies and hayfever. The baby's own immune system starts to become competent at about six months: consequently, the most vulnerable period for a child is between three and six months.

A study carried out in Finland showed that the children most likely to suffer from hayfever caused by birch pollen were those born in September, three months before the start of the birch pollen hayfever season. Other factors that make hayfever more likely are being male and being born prematurely.

PREGNANCY

Peak mother's health during pregnancy is vital to reduce the child's risk of suffering hayfever and allergy. Mothers who expose their children to a constant repetitive diet and high levels of pollution in air, food and water (e.g. cigarette smoke, chemical fumes, food additives, impure tap water), produce children that have a greater risk of allergy. The earlier in pregnancy the exposure occurs, the greater the risk of allergy problems.

INFANCY

Breast-feeding is very important to the developing infant because the antibodies in mother's milk help the baby fight infection as well as helping it to cope with an environment potentially full of allergic substances. Cow's milk is designed for baby cows; human milk is designed for human babies – consequently, mother's milk is much more easily digested by growing babies. Breast-fed babies therefore tend to grow better and also have a greater resistance to disease and infection.

WHAT FACTORS ARE LIKELY TO CAUSE INCREASED RISK OF HAYFEVER?

These have already been mentioned in various parts of the book; however, it is helpful to draw them all together into one list.

Heredity

Allergies, especially atopic allergies like hayfever, eczema and asthma, are very commonly inherited. The greater the degree of allergies in the families of both partners, the greater the risk that the children will suffer from allergies like hayfever.

In rearing livestock, farmers constantly select the fittest individuals from which to breed. For better or for worse, humans do not work to this plan and there is a slight tendency for the less fit members of the species to have more children, consequently increasing the incidence of their inherited diseases. However, nature compensates for this to some extent since patients with allergic disease tend to have a reduced fertility and, consequently, irrelevant of their wishes, they are less able to have children.

Adequate Intake of Vitamins and Minerals

Deficiencies of vitamins and minerals make the body more susceptible to allergies. Adequate amounts of vitamins and minerals and other nutrients are essential for good health. They are particularly important in allergic disease, since they help the body repair itself. During an allergic illness, the daily requirement of a specific vitamin, mineral or other nutrient may be dramatically increased.

Deficiencies of vitamins, minerals and other nutrients may occur because of four reasons. Either the diet may be deficient in these substances, or else there may be an interaction between the substances and food or bacteria in the gut. Assuming an adequate dietary intake and no interaction in the bowels, body levels may still be inadequate due to failure of absorption of the vitamins and minerals from the gut into the body, or alternatively the absorbed substances cannot be used, possibly because of a deficiency of a co-factor (a substance which is needed in order for nutrients to be absorbed or used properly).

Other Habits

Alcohol, smoking and drugs (prescribed or otherwise) all take their toll on the immune system and contribute to the total load of neotoxins.

General State of Health

This influences how much resistance a person has to allergic challenges, including hayfever. It is noticeable that some patients suffer from hayfever symptoms only when they are ill with some other condition.

Total Load of Neotoxins

This is a fundamental concept in environmental medicine. The state of the immune system is very strongly influenced by your total load of neotoxins. If your food and drink contain many additives and/or you are exposed to many chemicals and/or electromagnetic radiation and have a highly stressed lifestyle, then you are more likely to suffer an allergic problem. The higher your total load due to pollution of air, food and water, the greater the risk of allergy and hayfever.

Breast-Feeding

It is very important that, after birth, a baby is exclusively fed on breast milk with no cow's milk bottles at all and that the mother continues on her unpolluted, organic diet with spring water. Neotoxins from polluted food are concentrated into mother's milk. Ideally, weaning should be postponed until the baby is at least six months old. When weaning is started, food should be rotated (each food taken not more than once every three days).

If the baby has a bowel infection causing diarrhoea (and damage to the bowel wall), all food should be stopped and the baby should be given spring water only until the diarrhoea ceases.

Continuing Nutrition

This is the single most important factor that influences the development of allergy. Despite the extra cost, organic foods are very important for health. They contain the natural balance of proteins, carbohydrates and fats, vitamins and minerals and should be completely free of chemical contaminants, e.g. colourings, flavourings, other food additives, pesticides, petrochemicals and toxic metals.

HAYFEVER AND EXAMS

The peak age incidence of hayfever is in the late teens and the grass pollen season is in June and July. Consequently, large numbers of teenagers suffer hayfever symptoms at a time when they are taking important exams. In order to get the best results from the hayfever plan, read chapter 12 and decide which changes you need to make to your lifestyle at least three months before the hayfever season starts. If you haven't started by 1st April, then you may easily turn out to be an April Fool.

- Learn which techniques and therapies are most suitable for you. They may vary a little from year to year but generally when you find a plan that works, stick with it.
- If you do need to use prescribed drugs, take them exactly as directed before the symptoms begin.
- It is much more difficult to get rid of symptoms once the underlying hayfever process has started. You may need to use an antihistamine preparation. If this is the case, try to use a second generation product (see page 90) which is much less likely to cause sedation and drowsiness.
- Consult your teacher and advise the examining authorities of your hayfever.

In many cases, examination boards are able to make provision for students whose examination performance has been adversely affected by illness or hayfever. You will probably need some sort of certification from your doctor who will need to mention details of nature and severity of the hayfever symptoms, together with side effects such as sedation caused by prescribed medicines. It is also useful for the doctor to mention for how long the symptoms have occurred and how these may have affected the patient during the revision period immediately prior to the exam. In the worst possible scenario in which you are forced to miss an examination due to hayfever and/or the side effects of treatment, it may be possible for your doctor to issue a certificate which the examination board will accept as an aegrotat (literally, he/she is ill). In some cases, when there is suitable course work, this is accepted as a pass grade but it is very important to discuss this with the examination authorities well before the examination period.

Are There Any Ways to Modify the Examination Room?

Exams are usually taken in large airy halls with a considerable degree of ventilation (and likely entry of pollen). By special arrangement, it may be possible to modify the place in which the examination is taken in order to reduce the level of symptoms. Possible measures include:

* taking the exam in a small room in which the windows and doors are closed and an air filter has been left running overnight in order to remove suspended pollen grains
* by arrangement, it may be possible to take the examination at another centre where pollen levels are much lower, e.g. in seaside towns.

Pay attention to details. As you will have gathered from this book so far, single measures on their own are rarely completely successful. The most successful plan usually combines many different measures, each of which on their own may have only a limited effect, but the sum total causes a dramatic improvement.

15

The Future

At present, at least one in three of the population in the western world suffers from allergic reactions. However, the person-to-person variation in response to any selected neotoxin is very great. For some considerable time now, scientists have wondered why one individual is made ill by a neotoxin like alcohol or tobacco, whereas another individual of similar age, sex and physical characteristics can expose themself to such a neotoxin over many years and get away apparently unscathed.

This highly toxin-resistant man or woman is sometimes said to possess 'The Churchill Gene', a reference to the British statesman who smoked, drank, and drove his body to the limits with impunity until an advanced age.

The good news is that the emerging science of Environmental Medicine is starting to be able to explain why one person suffers from a disease whilst another similar person in identical conditions is unharmed – why one 43 year old woman, for example, who smokes 15 cigarettes a day, has three children and lives on a council estate, develops chronic bronchitis while her neighbour with a very similar life pattern does not.

In fact, the increased resistance to common neotoxins is not dependent on solely a single gene. As with most things in nature, the origin of this variation is multifactorial. It is particularly important to discover the reasons because once you know why someone becomes ill, you're at least half the way to finding a successful treatment or even avoiding the illness in the first place.

One of the fundamental tenets of Environmental Medicine is that there are two main reasons why people become ill:

- Genes inherited from parents are in some way defective and consequently essential enzymes and other vital cell proteins don't function properly.
- Some environmental factor, like diet, occupation, housing, hobbies or stress, damages these same enzyme systems and proteins and stops them from functioning properly.

Most illnesses are caused by some combination of the first and second reason, although the illness may not appear until a 'trigger factor' like a virus infection, massive exposure to chemicals, or an accident, shock or bereavement befalls the patient and depresses the immune system. Once the illness has started, it may often be difficult to return to full health because physical tissue damage may have occurred but sometimes this is largely reversible.

Increasingly, the effect of environmental factors like diet, occupation, housing, hobbies and stress on health are starting to become better appreciated. No doubt, by the end of the next decade, such questions about all these aspects of lifestyle will become a standard part of any serious medical consultation.

However, the most exciting ideas are emerging in the field of enzyme activity and the effect that damaged genes and environmental factors have on this activity. The enormous person-to-person variation in enzyme activity is now starting to be appreciated and Environmental Medicine doctors are correlating it with disease. This variation in enzyme activity explains why one person can drink half a bottle of whisky without becoming intoxicated, whereas another apparently similar person gets drunk after just half a glass of sherry.

As a general rule the young, the old, the pregnant and those already ill are most vulnerable to substances like alcohol although there are sometimes surprises. Occasionally, you will come across a woman in her sixties who is able to take large amounts of hard liquor due to a lifetime's regular drinking, whereas an apparently fit young man whom you might expect to have a high resistance to drink becomes unsteady on his feet after half a glass of sherry.

There is similar variation amongst smokers in the ability to cope with cigarette smoke. About one smoker in four does very badly and dies prematurely in their forties or fifties, whereas the other three have only a slightly reduced life expectancy. Most smokers dispute the health risk of their habit by relating stories of a relative or friend who reached an advanced age (like Churchill) despite drinking like a fish and smoking like a chimney. Unfortunately, they usually fail to realize that this enhanced survival is very much the exception to the rule and, had their friend (or Churchill) not smoked, he may easily have got to a hundred.

An idea that I am researching is a technique of classifying body biochemistry which I call 'chemotyping'. This is an advance on the well-recognized biological concepts of the genotype (the complement of genes that an individual is born with), and the phenotype (the physical appearance of an individual). The 'chemotype' is a useful way of expressing how well various enzyme systems work and it gives an indication of the resistance to disease.

The value of this system is that it helps the practitioner to identify patients most likely to suffer from specific diseases and even gives an indication of which treatment may work best.

Another very exciting field is the use of computer programmes in diagnosing allergy, analysing patients' lifestyles and pinpointing the toxins they may be exposed to. Research shows that people are more honest when giving information like smoking and drinking habits to a computer, which is seen as much less judgemental than a live doctor.

There is little doubt that, due to the amazing ability of Environmental Medicine to help a wide variety of modern illnesses caused by pollution of our food and water, it is only a matter of time until it becomes an integral part of every medical consultation. My only hope is that this revolution in medical care occurs over the next five years rather than taking 25 years.

APPENDIX: USA POLLEN CHART

This guide has been prepared in order to give you an idea of the likely pollen seasons for the plants causing hayfever and growing in your state. The timings are of necessity approximate since there will be individual variations in the pollen seasons from place to place within any individual state. This is due to different micro-environments, e.g. variations in temperature, shelter, rainfall and soil condition from place to place. As a general rule, the further north you go, the later the pollen season starts.

State	Jan Feb Mar Apr May Jun Jul Aug Sep Oct Nov Dec	Major sources of pollens and flowering season
Alabama		Trees Elm (Feb-March), Oak, Walnut (April), Pecan (April-May)
		Grasses Bermuda, Kentucky Blue (March-Nov), Johnson, Orchard, Red Top (April-Sept), Blue (April-Winter), Timothy (May-Sept)
		Weeds Ragweed (Mid Aug-End Oct)
Alaska		Trees No major problem
		Grasses Kentucky Blue, Red Top, Timothy (June-July)
		Weeds No major problem
Arizona		Trees No major problem
		Grasses Bermuda (Feb-Nov)
		Weeds Careless Weed (May-Sept)
Arkansas		Trees Elm (Feb-March), Oak (March-May), Pecan (April-May)
		Grasses Bermuda, Johnson (March-Nov), Kentucky Blue, Orchard, Red Top, Timothy (March-June)
		Weeds Ragweed (Mid August-Mid Oct)

California	▬▬▬▬▬	Trees	Elm (Feb-March), Cottonwood (Feb-April), Oak, Birch (Feb-May), Sycamore (March-May), Walnut (March-June), Olive (April-June)
	▬▬▬▬▬▬	Grasses	Bermuda, Brome, Red Top, Rye, Wild Oats (April-Oct)
	▬▬▬▬▬	Weeds	Pigweed (May-Oct), Sagebrush (July-Oct), Ragweed (July-Sept)
Colorado	▬▬▬▬	Trees	Elm (Feb-May), Cottonwood (April-May)
	▬▬▬▬▬	Grasses	Kentucky Blue (May-Sept)
	▬▬▬	Weeds	Kochia, Russian Thistle (July-Sept)
Connecticut	▬▬	Trees	Elm (April), Oak (May)
	▬▬▬	Grasses	Kentucky Blue, Orchard, Red Top, Timothy (End May-Mid July)
	▬	Weeds	Ragweed (Mid Aug-Mid Sept)
Delaware	▬▬	Trees	Elm (April), Oak (May)
	▬▬▬	Grasses	Kentucky Blue, Orchard, Red Top, Vernal (Mid May to July), Rye (June-July)
	▬▬▬	Weeds	Ragweed (Mid Aug-Oct)

State	Jan Feb Mar Apr May Jun Jul Aug Sep Oct Nov Dec	Major sources of pollens and flowering season
Dist of Columbia		**Trees** Elm (March-April), Oak (April-May) **Grasses** Kentucky Blue, Orchard, Red Top, Rye (May-July), Vernal (May-June), Timothy (June-July) **Weeds** Ragweed (Mid Aug-Mid Sept)
Florida		**Trees** Pecan (Dec-April), Oak, Pine (Feb-April) **Grasses** Bermuda, Johnson (April-Oct) **Weeds** Ragweed (July-Oct)
Georgia		**Trees** Elm (Feb-March), Oak (March-May) **Grasses** Kentucky Blue (March-July), Bermuda, Johnson (May-Oct) **Weeds** Ragweed (Aug-Oct)
Hawaii		**Trees** **Grasses** Low levels all pollen **Weeds**
Idaho		**Trees** No major problem **Grasses** Kentucky Blue, Red Top (May-Sept) **Weeds** Russian Thistle (June-Sept)

Illinois	▬▬▬▬	Trees	Elm (Feb-April), Oak (May)
	▬▬	Grasses	Kentucky Blue, Orchard, Red Top, Timothy, (Mid May-Mid July)
	▬▬	Weeds	Ragweed (Start Aug-End Sept)
Indiana	▬▬▬▬	Trees	Elm (Feb-March), Oak (April-May)
	▬▬	Grasses	Kentucky Blue, Orchard, Red Top, Timothy (May-June)
	▬▬	Weeds	Ragweed (Aug-Sept)
Iowa	▬▬▬	Trees	Elm, Walnut (March-April), Oak (April-May)
	▬▬	Grasses	Kentucky Blue, Orchard, Red Top, Timothy (May-June)
	▬	Weeds	Marsh Elder, Ragweed (Mid Aug-End Sept)
Kansas	▬▬▬	Trees	Elm (March), Oak (May)
	▬▬▬	Grasses	Kentucky Blue, Orchard, Red Top, Timothy (May-July)
	▬▬▬▬	Weeds	Kochia, Russian Thistle (July-Oct), Ragweed (Mid Aug-Mid Oct)
Kentucky	▬▬▬	Trees	Elm (Feb-March), Oak (April-May)
	▬▬▬	Grasses	Kentucky Blue, Timothy (May-July)
	▬▬	Weeds	Ragweed (Mid Aug-Start Oct)

State		Major sources of pollens and flowering season
Louisiana	Trees	Elm, Oak (Feb-April), Pecan (March-May)
	Grasses	Bermuda, Johnson (April-Dec)
	Weeds	March Elder, Ragweed (Aug-Nov)
Maine	Trees	Elm (April), Oak (May)
	Grasses	Kentucky Blue, Orchard, Red Top, Rye, Vernal (May to June), Timothy (May to July)
	Weeds	Ragweed (Mid Aug-Oct)
Maryland	Trees	Elm (March-April), Oak (April-May)
	Grasses	Kentucky Blue, Orchard, Red Top, Rye (May-July), Vernal (May-June), Timothy (June-July)
	Weeds	Ragweed (Mid Aug-Mid Sept)
Massachusetts	Trees	Ash, Elm, Hickory (April), Oak (May-June)
	Grasses	Foscue, Kentucky Blue, Orchard, Red Top, Timothy, Vernal (May-July)
	Weeds	Ragweed (Mid Aug-End of Sept)

Michigan	Trees	Elm (April), Oak (May)
	Grasses	Kentucky Blue, Orchard, Red Top, Timothy (May-July)
	Weeds	Ragweed (Mid Aug-Mid Sept)
Minnesota	Trees	Elm (April-May), Oak (May)
	Grasses	Kentucky Blue, Orchard, Red Top, Timothy (May-Aug)
	Weeds	Ragweed (Aug-Sept)
Mississippi	Trees	Elm, Pecan (March-April), Oak (April-May)
	Grasses	Bermuda, Johnson (April-Oct)
	Weeds	March Elder, Ragweed (Aug-Oct)
Missouri	Trees	Elm (March), Oak (May)
	Grasses	Kentucky Blue, Orchard, Red Top, Timothy (May-Aug)
	Weeds	Ragweed (Aug-End Sept)
Montana	Trees	No major problem in most areas
	Grasses	Kentucky Blue, Red Top (May-June)
	Weeds	Russian Thistle (July-Sept)

State	Jan Feb Mar Apr May Jun Jul Aug Sep Oct Nov Dec	Major sources of pollens and flowering season
Nebraska		Trees: Elm (March), Oak (May) Grasses: Kentucky Blue, Orchard, Red Top, Timothy (May-July) Weeds: Russian Thistle (July-Aug), Ragweed (Mid Aug-Oct)
Nevada		Trees: No major problem in most areas Grasses: Bermuda (March-Oct), Kentucky Blue, (May-July) Weeds: Russian Thistle (July-Sept), Sagebrushes (Aug-Sept)
New Hampshire		Trees: Elm (April), Oak (May) Grasses: Kentucky Blue, Orchard, Red Top, Rye, Timothy, Vernal (May-July) Weeds: Ragweed (Mid Aug-Sept)
New Jersey		Trees: Elm (March-April), Ash (April), Hickory (April-May), Oak (May) Grasses: Fescue, Kentucky Blue, Orchard, Red Top, Timothy (May-July) Weeds: Ragweed (Mid Aug-Sept)
New Mexico		Trees: No major problem Grasses: Bermuda (April-Aug) Weeds: Kochia, Russian Thistle (June-Sept)

New York	▬▬▬	Trees	Elm (April), Birch, Cottonwood (April-May), Oak (May)
	▬▬▬▬▬	Grasses	Fescue (May-June), Kentucky Blue, Orchard, Red Top (Mid May-July), Timothy (June-July)
	▬	Weeds	Ragweed (Mid Aug-Mid Sept)
North Carolina	▬▬▬	Trees	Elm (Feb-April), Oak (March-May)
	▬▬▬▬▬▬▬	Grasses	Bermuda, Johnson, Kentucky Blue, Orchard, Red Top, Timothy (March-Sept)
	▬▬▬	Weeds	Ragweed (Mid July-Start Oct)
North Dakota		Trees	No major problem
	▬▬▬	Grasses	Kentucky Blue (May-July)
	▬▬▬	Weeds	Kochia, Russian Thistle (June-Aug), Marsh Elder, Ragweed (July-Sept)
Ohio	▬▬	Trees	Elm, Sycamore (April), Oak (May)
	▬▬	Grasses	Fescue, Kentucky Blue, Orchard, Red Top, Timothy (Mid May-Mid July)
	▬	Weeds	Kochia (Aug), Ragweed (Aug-Mid Sept)
Oklahoma	▬▬▬	Trees	Elm (March-April), Walnut (April), Oak (May)
	▬▬▬▬	Grasses	Bermuda, Johnson, Kentucky Blue (May-Aug)
	▬▬▬	Weeds	Marsh Elder (Aug-Sept), Ragweed (End Aug-Oct)

State	Jan Feb Mar Apr May Jun Jul Aug Sep Oct Nov Dec	Major sources of pollens and flowering season
Oregon		**Trees** Alder, Birch (March-April), Walnut (May-June)
		Grasses Kentucky Blue, Timothy (May-Sept)
		Weeds Dock, Plantain (May-Sept), Lamb's Quarters, Pigweed (June-Sept), Russian Thistle (July-Sept)
Pennsylvania		**Trees** Elm (March-April), Birch, Oak, Sycamore, (April-May)
		Grasses Canadian Blue, Kentucky Blue, Orchard, Red Top, Timothy, Vernal (Mid May-Mid July)
		Weeds Ragweed (Mid Aug-Late Sept)
Rhode Island		**Trees** Elm (April), Oak (May)
		Grasses Kentucky Blue, Orchard, Red Top, Timothy, Vernal (Mid May-Mid July)
		Weeds Dock, Lamb's Quarters (July-Sept), Ragweed (Mid Aug-Mid Sept)
South Carolina		**Trees** Elm (April), Pecan (April-May), Oak (May)
		Grasses Bermuda, Johnson, Kentucky Blue (May-Sept)
		Weeds Ragweed (July-Oct)

South Dakota	Trees	No major tree problem
	Grasses	Kentucky Blue (May-July)
	Weeds	Kochia, Russian Thistle (June-Aug), Ragweed (July-Sept)
Tennessee	Trees	Elm (Feb-April), Pecan (April), Oak (April-May)
	Grasses	Bermuda, Johnson, Kentucky Blue (March-Nov)
	Weeds	Ragweed (Mid Aug-End October)
Texas	Trees	Elm (Feb-April)
	Grasses	Bermuda, Johnson, Kentucky Blue (Feb-Aug)
	Weeds	Ragweed (Late Aug-Start Oct)
Utah	Trees	Elder (April-May)
	Grasses	Kentucky Blue (May-July)
	Weeds	Kochia, Russian Thistle (July-Sept)
Vermont	Trees	Elm (April), Oak (May)
	Grasses	Kentucky Blue, Orchard, Red Top, Rye, Timothy, Vernal (May-July)
	Weeds	Ragweed (Mid Aug-Mid Sept)

State	Jan	Feb	Mar	Apr	May	Jun	Jul	Aug	Sep	Oct	Nov	Dec	Major sources of pollens and flowering season
Virginia													Trees: Elm, Maple (Feb-April), Oak, Hickory (April-May) Grasses: Bermuda, Johnson, Kentucky Blue, Orchard, Red Top, Rye, Timothy, Vernal (May-July) Weeds: Ragweed (Start Aug-Start October)
Washington													Trees: No major problem in most places Grasses: Kentucky Blue (May-Sept), Timothy (June-July) Weeds: Plantain, Russian Thistle (June-Sept), Marsh Elder, Ragweed (Aug-Sept)
West Virginia													Trees: Elm, Sycamore (April), Walnut (April-May), Oak (May) Grasses: Johnson, Kentucky Blue, Orchard, Red Top, Timothy (May-July) Weeds: Plantain (May-July), Ragweed (Mid Aug-Late September)
Wisconsin													Trees: Elm (April), Oak (May) Grasses: Kentucky Blue, Orchard, Red Top, Timothy (June-July) Weeds: Ragweed (Start Aug-End Sept)
Wyoming													Trees: No major problem in most places Grasses: Kentucky Blue (May-July) Weeds: Kochia, Russian Thistle (July-Sept)

FURTHER READING

Davies, Robert and Ollier, Susan, *Allergy, the Facts*, Oxford University Press, 1989

Mackarness, Dr Richard, *Allergies*, Thorsons, 1981

Mackarness, Dr Richard, *Not All In The Mind*, Pan Books, 1976

Mackay, Ian, *Rhinitis*, Royal Society of Medicine Services, 1989

Payne, Mark, *Superhealth: The Complete Environmental Medicine Health Plan*, Thorsons, 1992

Payne, Mark, *Superhealth in a Toxic World*, HarperCollins USA, 1992

Thomson, C. Neil, Kirkwood, M. Eve, Lever, S. Rosemary, *Handbook of Clinical Ecology*, Blackwell Scientific Publications, 1990

FURTHER INFORMATION

The author can be contacted at the following address:

Dr Mark Payne
20 Coppice Walk
Cheswick Green
Solihull
West Midlands
B90 4HY
Tel: 0546 2186

INDEX

DIETS TO HELP ASTHMA AND HAYFEVER

Roger Newman Turner

Asthma and hayfever can be made worse by eating certain foods, but there are also nutritional guidelines that you can follow to help *manage* the condition. This book explains:

- why some people are prone to asthma or hayfever
- how to cut down on mucus-forming foods
- how to increase your intake of protective vitamins and minerals

It includes basic diets to help control the condition and specific diets for more acute symptoms.

Roger Newman Turner is a leading naturopath, osteopath and acupuncturist. He has many years' experience treating a wide range of conditions and runs practices in Harley Street, London and Letchworth, Hertfordshire, UK.